THE *X* OF PSYCHOLOGY

LONDON : HUMPHREY MILFORD
OXFORD UNIVERSITY PRESS

The X of Psychology

AN ESSAY ON THE PROBLEM OF THE SCIENCE OF MIND

BY

PHILLIPS MASON

Professor of Philosophy, Bowdoin College

CAMBRIDGE, MASSACHUSETTS

HARVARD UNIVERSITY PRESS

1940

PRINTED AT THE HARVARD UNIVERSITY PRESS
CAMBRIDGE, MASSACHUSETTS, U.S.A.

TO THE MEMORY OF

PAUL NATORP

PREFACE

THE X OF PSYCHOLOGY as a study in the foundation of psychology was planned and sketched in part many years ago. Parts of the original sketch are included in Chapter III. Some years later the plan was revised so that it might include an account of my general philosophical position without which the position taken with regard to the foundation of psychology seemed unintelligible. The earlier part of Chapter II was then written. More recently the work has been put together and arranged in its present form. It was at first intended to include a more detailed account of several phases of the subject, especially of the relation of psychology to logic, to ethics, to aesthetics, and to ontology. To do so it would have been necessary to enlarge the work by three or four chapters, but such an addition would have upset its balance by giving too much space to matters not central to the subject. As it stands now, after the introductory chapter, the work divides naturally into two parts. In the first part, Chapter II, my philosophical position in the form of a theory of knowledge or theory of truth is developed. In the second part, Chapters III, IV, and V, the foundation of psychology is worked out on the basis of the more general theory of the first part, and in this second part the content and method of psychology as well as its place in the field of knowledge are defined.

My point of view is based on the Critical Philosophy of Kant, and is largely the result of a study of his thought. I have sought to develop the objective side of his teaching, and at the same time to find the proper place for the subjective. I have treated his synthetic logic as primary and fundamental, and I have regarded the subjective or mental factor as secondary and in no wise central to his logic. My interpretation of his thought has made it possible to eliminate all suggestion of subjective idealism or of ontological idealism. It has meant Kant without Fichte and Hegel. Since ample suggestion is given in Kant as to the secondary place of the subjective, my interpretation has also meant Kant without the interpretations of Fries and his school. I am not a strict follower of Kant; I have tried rather to work out those sides of his philosophy which seem to me to have permanent value and so to throw light on many of the problems of the present. My work is, however, not merely the product of my study of Kant. I owe much to many other thinkers, particularly to Plato and Descartes, as also in lesser degree to Aristotle, Leibniz, and Hume. To Cohen and Natorp of the Marburg School I am greatly indebted for my understanding of Plato, Descartes, and Kant. Natorp originally suggested to me that I undertake research along the lines carried out in this work.

It may seem to the reader that most of what I have said is not Kantian, and that my mode of expression sounds very little like the language of Kant. The emphasis on truth with knowledge as its second dimension, the significance of relation, as also the relational theory of truth, my conception of the logical core, logical idealism, and epistemological idealism, including the dynamic conception of truth, do not at first sight suggest anything in Kant; yet I think they all bear out important phases of his philosophy. The treatment of mind as consciousness and as determinable only after the determination of its object is clearly in Kant, as is also much of my outline of mind (Chapter V). Furthermore, the ego-content theory, as opposed to any such theory as that of behaviorism or even as opposed to the content theory, is Kantian, but the transformation of the ego-content theory into the awareness-unity theory is a development which goes beyond Kant. The fuller definition of mind as I have developed it, the conceptions of unity, awareness, limitation of content, and truth as the content of mind, and the more general conception of the place of mind in truth, are to be sure further developments of Kant's thought, but not out of tune with his fundamental teaching. That in the connecting, massing, and changing of the content of mind the content may not be limited to content of present time, and that there may be sequences in the content which are not sequences in time, may seem strange; and the reconstructive method which was first suggested by Cohen and Natorp may be regarded as extreme and unreasonable. But all the conceptions which I have put forward are appropriate to the Critical Philosophy, and form, I feel sure, genuine additions to it. The reference to the *Gestalt* psychology (Chapter V) as coming nearer than any other psychology to my outline does not mean that it is by any means an adequate psychology; it is valuable largely because it lays stress on relations and might well be expanded into a much broader conception. I hope that in considering the various conceptions and theories which I have endeavored to explain the reader will judge of their value in the light of the whole body of theory with regard to truth and mind, both as it stands in Kant and as it has been developed since Kant.

Many of the ideas and many phases of the thought of my teachers in philosophy are reflected in this work. I was fortunate in being able to study at Harvard with five great teachers – Palmer, James, Royce, Santayana, and Münsterberg – and to begin my study of philosophy under their guidance. They opened up to me the world of philosophy and aroused in me a vital interest in its problems. I was also fortunate in studying with Cohen and Natorp at Marburg; to them I owe more than to any of my other teachers my fundamental point of view and my conception of the primary philosophical problems. Although I probably should not be counted a strict adherent of the Marburg School, much of their thought, particularly that of Natorp relative to the problem of psychology, runs through this work. Two other teachers who have left their traces in my thought should be mentioned – Professor Henri Bergson and the late President Thomas Case. I am appreciative too of much that I have learned from Professor Edwin B. Holt, both in discussion and from his writings. There are many others, teachers, colleagues, friends, and thinkers whose works I have read, from whom I have received various ideas and suggestions, but it would be impossible to refer to them all. I am most grateful to Professor Holt and to three colleagues here at Bowdoin

College, Professor Charles T. Burnett, Professor Newton P. Stallknecht, and Professor Fritz C. A. Kölln, who have gone over my manuscript with great care and have offered many valuable suggestions with regard both to the thought expressed and to the form of exposition. Professor C. H. Rieber also read my manuscript and made valuable comment on it. Many thanks are due to Miss Edith R. Collins for the great care she has taken in preparing the work for publication.

PHILLIPS MASON

Bowdoin College
Brunswick, Maine

CONTENTS

THE *X* OF PSYCHOLOGY

CHAPTER I

THE PROBLEM OF PSYCHOLOGY

THIS WORK is not a work in psychology but on psychology. It asks what psychology is, it seeks to determine its proper problem, and its appropriate method. What is the psychological *x*, and how can it be determined?

Three phases of the psychological problem at once suggest themselves for consideration. These are the problems of the content of psychology, of its relation to the other sciences, and of its methods. A consideration of any one of these phases involves the very foundations of knowledge. Psychology is said to be the science of mind. Among the various definitions of mind, mind is found characterized as consciousness and again as behavior. Such basic concepts as consciousness and behavior cannot be made clear and definite without careful analysis. Analysis cannot be made without the use of concepts which are more fundamental, and these lead back ultimately to the fundamental categories of knowledge. A definition of mind, or a consideration of the merits of consciousness and behavior as definitions of mind, thus implies reference to the first principles of truth.

A consideration of the relation of psychology to the other sciences points in the same direction. According to one view of this relation, psychology is contrasted with and set over against the other sciences. It is said to be a subjective science as opposed to the physical sciences. These sciences have to do with the outer world, with phenomena as determined in space–time, while psychology is concerned with the inner world, with phenomena so far as they are not in space–time but are related to a non-spatial subject or mind. According to another view, psychology has a definite place in the gamut of the sciences. It is thought to be based on physical science and is more especially connected with biology. Just as general physics is based on logic and mathematics, and biology is thought to be based on physics, so psychology is thought to be based on biology or is even regarded as a branch of biology. The relative merits of these two views imply reference to a full perspective of the sciences and of knowledge, and this means reference to the whole structure of truth.

Furthermore, the content of psychology cannot be determined without reference to the content of the other sciences. The definition of the subject matter of the other sciences may affect the definition of the subject matter of psychology, and vice versa. Psychology may be dependent upon the other sciences or the other sciences may be dependent upon psychology. Such questions can only be settled in the light of the whole system of truth.

Again, a consideration of the methods of psychology leads back to fundamentals. Much has been said as to the relative merits of two methods of description of mental phenomena. According to one method the mind is studied on the basis of its observation of itself, and according to the other the signs of mind in the activities of the organism are used as clues to the nature of mind. The former method is called the method of self-observation or introspection, and its peculiar characteristic lies in the fact that only one observer can observe any one mind or any one case of a mental phenomenon. The latter method is called the method of external observation, the signs of mind being open to all observers, as is the case with the observation of all biological and physical phenomena. It is claimed that the peculiar characteristic of introspection makes it inaccurate or less accurate than the method of external observation, which falls in line with the method of observation used in physical science. The question naturally arises as to whether the method of introspection should be given up in favor of the more accurate and more fully developed method of external observation, or whether it should be retained as an auxiliary to the method of external observation and possibly as having value in itself because even inaccurate knowledge, knowledge not measuring up to the highest ideal of scientific accuracy, is still knowledge and has its place in the whole system of knowledge. The question of scientific accuracy versus completeness of knowledge can only be settled by reference to the fundamental principles of knowledge or the whole structure of truth. The whole question of methods depends upon the question of content and of the relation of psychology to the other sciences. The interest may be centered in the content of psychology, or in its methods, or in its relation to the field of knowledge; but whatever phase of the problem of psychology is considered, this problem inevitably leads back to and involves the consideration of the fundamental principles and system of truth and so of the whole field of knowledge.

The procedure in this work will then be as follows: First, the general nature and structure of truth will be considered; secondly, mind or the object of psychology; thirdly, the relation of mind to truth and of psychology to the other sciences; and finally, the content and method of psychology.

Stated more briefly, the problem as to the nature of psychology is the problem as to what the true problem of psychology is. It is the problem of the problem of psychology. And the problem of the problem of psychology is a problem of knowledge, a problem to be solved by reference to the structure of truth. First, then, as to truth.

CHAPTER II

TRUTH

OF THE VARIOUS THEORIES OF TRUTH only two give a suggestion as to its structure, and these are the correspondence and coherence theories. According to the correspondence [1] theory, a thought is said to be true if it corresponds to or represents the real facts. The thought that a molecule of water is made up of a certain arrangement of atoms of oxygen and hydrogen is true, if the real physical molecule of water is so made up. The thought must agree with the object which it is intended to represent: there must be, as Joachim says, a "one–one relation" [2] between them, so that the thought embodies the nature of the thing in every detail.

It is essential to this theory that the facts, objects, or things be regarded as distinct from the thoughts which represent them, otherwise a correspondence between them would be impossible. On the other hand it is just as essential that the facts, etc., should not be absolutely separated from the thoughts, for if they were it is hard to see how a correspondence between them could be determined. In the case of the molecule of water, if the real molecule were treated as a thing in the physical world and the thought of the molecule as a sort of thing in the thought-world, and if the physical world were not allowed to enter the thought-world, then the thought of the molecule could not be compared with the real molecule and made to agree with it. To avoid this absolute separation the facts must be brought in touch with the thoughts without at the same time becoming identical with them. It is usual therefore to suppose that a basis for the facts is given in perception. If the molecule itself does not appear in perception, at least facts directly connected with it and from which its

[1] Sir William Hamilton, *Lectures on Metaphysics and Logic* (Edinburgh and London, 1859–60), IV, 63; Harold Henry Joachim, *The Nature of Truth* (Oxford, 1906), pp. 7–30.

[2] Joachim, p. 9.

nature can be inferred are perceived and compared with the thoughts. Thus the dualism of facts and thoughts is maintained by allowing the facts either directly or indirectly to be given. As given, the facts are distinguished from the thoughts, and form a sort of fact-world independent of the thoughts, and yet as given they serve as a standard to which the thoughts must conform.

There are, however, two difficulties with this theory. In the first place the connection between those facts which do not appear in perception and those which do is not accounted for by the correspondence of the thoughts with the facts. Some other principle is needed as the ground for the inference from the given facts to those beyond; and this principle is really presupposed by the correspondence theory, because without such inference the agreement between the thoughts and the facts not directly perceived could not be established. In defense of the theory it might be said that, though the correspondence cannot be established without the inference, truth consists only in the correspondence of the thoughts with the facts. But a theory which does not fully explain how truth is determined is hardly an adequate theory of truth. If the molecule were given directly in perception, the agreement of the thought with the molecule would offer a sufficient explanation; but as long as an inference from the perception to the molecule is necessary, and as long as an error in that inference is just as fatal as an error in the agreement of the thought with the fact, the basis of the inference forms an essential part of the theory of truth.

Then, secondly, it is questionable whether the assumption can be maintained that facts and thoughts are distinct. There are two ways in which the fact and the thought can be related. Either the fact and the thought are qualified each separately by a content, or they are qualified by one identical content. For instance, the fact given in perception that water is transparent is either distinct from the thought which corresponds to it or identical with the thought, so far as both are qualified by the content that water is transparent. If the first alternative is assumed, that the fact and the thought are qualified separately, and if the correspondence is perfect so that the content of the thought is exactly like the content of the fact, then the two contents, being exactly alike, are really identical. This first alternative leads to the second, and if the second alternative is assumed, then with identity of content correspondence is out of the question.[3] The objection might be raised that beyond the content in question the fact-world and the thought-world are distinct, and that therefore the content as qualifying each of those worlds need not be regarded as identical but as two distinct but like contents. But if truth consists in correspondence, it consists in a correspondence between a thought and a fact irrespective of what lies beyond in the fact-world or in the thought-world. And if an attempt is made to go further than the content of the fact and the thought, to explore the fact-world and the thought-world beyond, then, barring error, the same situation will result, namely a correspondence between the content of thoughts and facts; and the correspondence will again be shown to be impossible because of the identity of content of the supposedly distinct facts and thoughts. The dualism of fact and thought can then hardly be the basis of a theory of truth.

In sharp contrast with the correspondence theory, the coherence [4] theory makes no dualistic assumption and sets up no standard connected with facts given in perception, but aims first of all to show how a content is placed in the larger whole to which it belongs. A content is true, according to Joachim, as belonging to a "significant whole," and a "significant whole" is a whole "such that all its constituent elements reciprocally involve one another, or reciprocally determine one another's being as contributory features in a single concrete meaning. The elements thus cohering constitute a whole which may be said to control the reciprocal adjustments of its elements, as an end controls its constituent

[3] Joachim, *The Nature of Truth*, p. 25; Edwin B. Holt, *The Concept of Consciousness* (London, 1914), p. 35.

[4] Joachim, pp. 64–121; Bernard Bosanquet, *Logic* (2nd ed., Oxford, 1911), II, 263–294; Francis Herbert Bradley, *Essays on Truth and Reality* (Oxford, 1914), pp. 202–244.

means." [5] "The systematic coherence of such a whole is expressed most adequately and explicitly in the system of reasoned knowledge which we call a science or a branch of philosophy." [6] The truth of the molecule can only be found in its coherence or connection with other factors in a "whole" such that the "whole" determines the parts. "The coherence — if we call it a form — is a form which through and through interpenetrates its materials; and they — if we call them materials — are materials which retain no inner privacy for themselves in independence of the form." [7] In other words, a true content belongs to a group of contents, which contents in some way form a whole that in turn penetrates the contents and conditions their nature.

The value of this theory lies in its making truth relational. That means that truth does not consist of isolated entities but is essentially connected or coherent. A true content belongs in a context; a molecule as a factor in truth has a place in a connected system. And it is in reasoned knowledge, in science and philosophy, where particular truths and contents are closely interwoven, that the relational character of truth fully reveals itself.

There are, however, two unfortunate implications in the coherence theory as stated by Joachim. If the content is determined by the whole it is implied that there is no truth short of the whole. As he says, the "universal judgment" that 3 squared equals 9 is "hypothetical," and a "hypothetical judgment" involves a "categorical basis," and he makes the categorical basis "that sphere of being which the science in question expresses in the whole system of its reasoning." [8] The "categorical basis" is therefore the "whole" and only in the whole is the genuine truth to be found.[9] Propositions made by science with regard to the molecule of water would then not be true because they are not referred to the whole physical

[5] Joachim, *The Nature of Truth*, p. 66.
[6] Joachim, p. 68.
[7] Joachim, p. 77.
[8] Joachim, p. 96.
[9] Bertrand Russell, *Philosophical Essays* (London and New York, 1910), pp. 150–169.

system, and many of the so-called truths of science would not be valid. To demand a categorical or absolute basis of truth is really to do violence to its relative character. Science and philosophy may aim at the whole, but what they find by the way may be "significant." A content may be understood by reference to its context, without full knowledge of the system of its context. The problem of the whole is a more special problem of truth, and it is unfortunate that this concept should be introduced in connection with a theory otherwise as suggestive as the coherence theory.

The second implication is no less serious. The coherence is said to be a form "which interpenetrates its materials"; and allows them no "inner privacy." So far as this means that all material or content is coherent in the sense of being relational no objection can be made, but if it means that the larger relations or connections determine all the detail of the content then it is questionable. If the larger relations determine all contents then one content because of these larger relations would imply another content or all of the contents. In other words, knowledge of one content would make it possible to reason by implication to any other content, and the whole system of truth would be absolutely compact. No room would be left for contents which might be irrelevant to one another, and no content could give rise to any truth from its own nature. All relations between contents would be relations of mutual implication, and the various contents would have no relative independence. The relations of the content to the whole and of one content to another are too narrowly conceived by Joachim. There must be room for all types of relation, both independent and dependent, external and internal, if truth is to be conceived as truth and not as some special kind of truth.

The coherence theory may therefore be acceptable as a theory that truth is a system of relations, that it is not a system of disconnected truths but a coherent and interrelated body of truth. Science and philosophy may aim at the whole of truth and the best examples of truth may be found in closely reasoned systems of knowledge, but in any conception of the general structure of truth the "concept of the whole" and the concept of the "mutual implication" of the contents must not be made paramount.

If truth is to be regarded as a system of relations then a serious objection may be brought against this theory. It may be said that if truth is regarded as a structure, a connected or relational system, no place is left for error. Truth plays the part of the world of things or facts, and only by the introduction of thoughts over against the facts can any account of error be given. The correspondence theory regards the world of facts as a standard to which true thoughts conform and to which erroneous thoughts do not conform; through the dualism of facts and thoughts, it can easily explain error as a divergence of thoughts from the standard facts: whereas the coherence theory, not being dualistic, not admitting of any factor such as thought to play off against the true relational system, offers nothing through which to explain error. The objection seems to be a good one, and the coherence theory as a theory of truth seems to need by way of supplement the correspondence theory as a theory of error.

Undoubtedly the coherence theory is concerned with the positive structure of truth — it says that the content of truth is relational; and when the concept of the whole and the idea that coherence is a form determining all contents are eliminated, it offers a basis for a positive theory of truth to which it is difficult to make objection. But can its neglect of the negative side of truth be supplemented by the correspondence theory? By identifying the fact-world of the correspondence theory with the relational system of the coherence theory the first difficulty with the correspondence theory might be overcome, but hardly the second difficulty. The relational system might offer a sufficient basis for the inference from the facts given in perception to those beyond, but the identity of the true thoughts with the facts in the relational system would interfere with the dualism necessary to the correspondence theory. Of course identity might be admitted in the case of true thoughts and divergence in case of erroneous thoughts. But if the thought-world were given a separate status in order to explain error, that same status would have to hold when *true* thoughts were concerned, and this has been shown not to be possible. If a dualism is assumed at all, it must cover all cases — when the thoughts are true as well as when false. The dualism of the correspondence theory is therefore fatal to it, and yet it is probably because of the ease with which error is explained by this dualism that the correspondence theory has stood its ground so long. In spite of its failure as a theory, it does, however, suggest that something more than the positive structure of truth is needed to account for error. A dualism need not be involved, but at least some further complication beyond the mere relational system of the coherence theory is necessary. The correspondence theory cannot therefore supplement the coherence theory by attaching itself to the latter, but it can help to bring to light the incompleteness of that theory.

The foregoing criticism of these two theories leads then to the acceptance of the coherence theory in so far — and in so far only — as it makes truth relational, and to the rejection of the correspondence theory except in so far as it includes error as a factor in the theory of truth. As a result, truth may be regarded as a coherent or relational system, *provided* some place for error can be found which is consistent with such a system.

Before the theory of truth is further developed along the lines here suggested, the intuitional theory of truth ought to be mentioned. This theory brings out the direct relation of the mind to truth: the mind is said to take in the truth by immediate relation to it. Knowledge of it "consists in intuiting, in having a direct perception of, reality." [10] The theory centers in the relation of the truth to the mind and tells nothing as to the structure of truth itself. Descartes says that in attaining truth our ideas should be so "clear and distinct" [11] that they cannot be doubted, and that "obscure

[10] Joseph Alexander Leighton, *Man and the Cosmos* (New York, 1922), p. 51.

[11] René Descartes, *Discours de la Méthode,* Precept no. 1 (Œuvres, edited by Charles Adam and Paul Tannery, Paris, 1897–1910, vol. VI).

propositions" should be reduced to simpler ones and the mind should start with the "intuition" of those propositions which are "most simple" and then attempt "to ascend to the knowledge of all the others," [12] each proposition then being clearly apprehended by the mind. This procedure makes "clearness and distinctness" the criterion of truth; but such a criterion is distinctly subjective, and nothing is suggested as to what the truth might be over and above its relation to the mind. The theory is therefore very inadequate as a theory of truth, yet it does suggest the importance of the relation of truth to the mind if truth is to be determined at all. Some contact with the world of truth, some apprehension or awareness of it, is necessary in order that there be knowledge. Though nothing is suggested by this theory as to the structure of truth, it does emphasize the fact that a beginning must be made somewhere, that some starting point is necessary in the pursuit of truth.

The importance of the problem of error and of the question as to the starting point in the determination of truth will appear after consideration is given to the coherent or relational structure of truth. To understand truth as a system of relations it will first be necessary to consider the nature of relations. What is relation? And how do relations hang together to form a system of truth?

Royce defines relation with respect to the objects or terms related. He says that "relations in which any object stands are characters that are viewed as belonging to it when it is considered with explicit reference to, that is, as in ideal or real company with another object, or with several other objects." A relation is then "a character that an object possesses as a member of a collection, . . . and which . . . would not belong to that object, were it not such a member." [13] This definition makes a relation a character of objects, it is a kind of attribute of its terms. This view of rela-

[12] Descartes, *Regulae ad Directionem Ingenii*, Rule 5 (Œuvres, Adam and Tannery, vol. x).

[13] Josiah Royce, "The Principles of Logic," in *Encyclopaedia of the Philosophical Sciences*, edited by Wilhelm Windelband and Arnold Ruge, English edition by Sir Henry Jones (London, 1913), I, 96.

tion is the view most naturally taken by the human mind. The mind thinks primarily in terms of objects, and relations seem secondary to objects. The center of gravity lies in the terms and relations are relative to the terms. This view is unsatisfactory because it tells us very little as to the character of relation beyond the fact that in some way a relation involves terms; what the relation is beyond the terms is not clear. The recognition that a relation is not just an addendum to its terms, but that it is something to be reckoned with beyond the terms, has led to another view of relation.

This second view is stated by Spaulding. He begins by quoting Royce's definition,[14] but he later makes it clear that relations are of equal importance with terms. He says that "neither 'term' nor 'relation' is logically prior to the other." [15] The relation cannot then be treated as an attribute of its terms, it is an entity to be kept distinct from the terms although it must relate them. It is indefinable and something *sui generis.* Even this view tells us very little about relation, but it is important in that it recognizes that relation cannot occupy a subordinate place.

If the first view tends to subordinate the relation to its term, the second view may easily tend to make the relation too independent of its terms. To be a relation, the relation must relate, and the connection between the relation and its terms must be clear without loss to the relation of its full character.

A third view is therefore here offered which aims to supplement the other two views and to give a fuller foundation to relation as the fundamental character of truth. According to this view:

(1) A relation is a unity or synthesis or connection, not an isolated entity or quality. Its function is to unite, to make coherent, to bind, to bring together.

It may be said that to call a relation a unity or synthesis is merely to say a relation is a relation. It is true that it cannot

[14] Edward Gleason Spaulding, *The New Rationalism* (New York, 1918), p. 21.

[15] Spaulding, p. 410.

be reduced to anything else and is therefore indefinable, but its characterization as a unity or synthesis is here given only to bring out its primary function as a phase of its general character.

(2) The unity of a relation is specific, that is, every relation has definite character.

The unity is not unity in general or something distinct from the specific character of the relation but it is the unity brought about through the particular nature of the relation in question. For instance, in the causal relation or in the relation *at-a-distance-from,* being *the-cause-of* and being *at-a-distance-from* are not separate functions from the unity. The unity is expressed in being *the-cause-of,* or being *at-a-distance-from.* In other words, the general unity and the specific unity are not separate functions but phases of one function.

(3) A relation implies terms. The unity of a relation is a unity of a plurality. It unites or connects something with something. The members of the plurality are generally called the terms of the relation. There may be two, three, four, or any number of terms to a relation; there may possibly be only one term, as in the relation *a is identical with a.*

The terms are the terminals of the relation, and without them the relation would not be complete. If a relation had no terms it would not relate, that is, it would not perform its proper function of unifying or connecting.

(4) A relation involves direction or sense. The unity of a relation of two terms links one term with the other, or the other with the one.

In the example *a is the cause of b,* the direction in the relation is from *a* to *b.* Even in the relation *b is different from a,* the direction is from *a* to *b,* and if it be said that it is also true that *a is different from b,* the direction is from *b* to *a.* These are really two distinct relations of difference. It would not be accurate to regard the relation of difference as a unity of *a* and *b,* as if the unity were a sort of grouping of *a* and *b,* or as if difference were a sort of entity between *a* and *b* such that one might run from *a* to *b* or *b* to *a* through difference. One term is always referred to the other term. In relations which involve more than two terms the direction would still be involved, though in a more complex way. Direction as involved in relation is not a mere matter of the movement of the mind from one term to the other, but it is a definite factor in the structure of relation.

It may now be asked how relations fit together to form a system of truth, and what bearing each of the three views of relation outlined above may have on the theory of truth. As a result of the criticism of the coherence theory it may be said that while truth is a connected system it is not necessary to conceive it only in the light of the whole. As expressed in propositional form, truth is made up of many propositions, though the propositions which express it are connected and interrelated. Truth is not just whole and not mere part, but an interrelation of many relations. Relations then must do justice to this connective and synthetic character of truth, and if truth is a system of relations it must not do violence to the nature of relation.

If the first view of relation be regarded as the foundation of truth, the view that a relation is "a character that an object possesses as a member of a collection . . . ," then the system of truth is a system of the attributes of terms or things belonging to a group. The unity of the system would then lie in the unity of the group and not in the connections made by the relations. The relations would not perform their proper function in the system of truth, they would not be anything essential to it. The system of truth might as well be called a system of things having qualities or attributes. The unifying character of relation and the specific character of relation as relating are not brought out. It might further be pointed out that the group is a kind of relation of the things or terms, and that therefore relation is really presupposed as the foundation of this view. But the relations referred to are not identical with the relation of the group; they belong to the things in the group; the unity and the relations are kept apart. In short, this conception of truth as based upon the first view of relation does not account for the unity of the system of truth through relations, and it treats these relations as mere qualities of the terms in the system. The core of the world of truth is to be found in the terms or things, to which is added a halo of unity in the conception of the group. The relations being secondary to the terms, this conception of truth may well be called the terminal theory of truth. This theory of truth with its emphasis on terms is hardly a theory of truth as a system of relations. Apart from its being an unsatisfactory view of relation, it can hardly be said to give adequate foundation to the coherence theory of truth as essentially a connective or synthetic theory.

The second view of relation, according to Spaulding, makes relation of equal importance with its terms. It is neither an attribute of its terms nor subordinate to them, it stands out as a distinct entity. A system of truth as based upon this view of relation would be a system of terms and relations and might be called the terminal-relational theory of truth. If the relation is of equal importance with the terms and stands out as a distinct entity there is a danger that the relations may become too independent. In an analysis of the proposition *a causes b*, it may be pointed out that there are three distinct factors involved, *a*, *b*, and *cause*, and that *cause* (like *a* or *b*) may be treated as a sort of entity in itself, but which may be brought into connection with *a* and *b* so far as it performs the function of relating them. No doubt the specific character of the relation, *cause*, may be distinguished from *a* and *b*, but it is questionable whether *cause* means anything as a relation if it does not relate. Russell distinguishes between "a relation in itself and a relation actually relating," but he points out that the distinctive character of the "relation actually relating" lies in the unity of the proposition which expresses the relation.[16] The real danger would then seem to be that of separating the specific character of the relation from its unity. Just as terms are said to have being, so it is easy to think of the relations having being along with and beside the terms. The relations are then being treated along with the terms as if they were all terms in the analytical

[16] Bertrand Russell, *The Principles of Mathematics*, I (Cambridge, 1903), 49–50.

relation of difference. But to reduce a relation to a term in another relation is not to explain relation. The whole difficulty may be avoided by considering relation in its proper function, that is, as a relation of terms. The unit of truth as a system of relations and terms cannot, so far as relations go, be a bare relation; it can only be a relation as relating terms, that is, a relating relation.

The adherents of this view, however, might avoid this difficulty by admitting that there can be no bare relations only relating relations, and yet maintain that truth is made up of terms and relations. They might not allow any relations subsisting by themselves, but still regard relations as not identifiable with terms. Here a serious question arises. Even if the relations which help to make up the body of truth are relating relations, it may still be asked, do the terms always stand in relation? or may they subsist independently? If the terms subsist by themselves and the relations do not, then the terms would seem to have greater importance than the relations. To give them greater importance is probably not the intention of the second view of relation, but rather, to regard terms and relations as of equal importance.

What, then, are terms? A pine tree might be said to be a term when considered in relation to the soil or to the atmosphere, or the planet Venus might be said to be a term in the solar system. But both the pine tree and the planet Venus are not merely terms, because they are also very complicated systems of relations of terms. Any unit in relation to another unit may be a term to the relation, but at the same time it may be itself a very intricate complex of relations. If the pine tree or the planet Venus is a complicated system of relations of terms, the terms may be again systems of relations of further terms, and those relations of still further terms, and so on. But in order to rescue the terms, or some terms, from being relations, it may be inquired whether there are any ultimate terms which are not relations. Russell says, "There are terms which can never occur except as terms; such are points, instants, colours, sounds, bits of matter, and generally terms of the kind of which existents consist."[17] The "terms of the kind of which existents consist" is not definite in reference, but the other examples are specific and refer to three different fields of truth: "points" and "instants" to mathematics, the sensations of "colours" and "sounds" to psychology, and "bits of matter" to physical science. The pine tree and the planet Venus are said to be made up of "bits of matter," of atoms or of electrons and protons. Though the electrons and protons may be the lowest units which up to the present time physical science has suggested, there is probably no valid reason for assuming that these units are not systems of relations; and the same may be said of any further units of nature which science may later suggest. The sensations of "colours" and "sounds" might at first seem to be ultimate terms in the field of perception. But if a sensation in the field of perception cannot be further analyzed by the perceiving mind, it does not follow that the sensation is not itself a relation or a system of relations. If the mind cannot break it up into components it may still be made up of components and therefore be relational. As for the "points" and "instants" it is difficult to separate them from their relations in space and time. Should a point be regarded as a division of a line into two parts, or an instant a division of time into two parts? The point would be clearly a relation between the two parts of the line and the instant a relation between the two parts of time. Should a point be regarded as a position? It might possibly be said to be a term and not a relation, but it could mean nothing except as a position in a relational system, in space, and therefore it could have no independent subsistence. The point as a position is essentially internal to the system of relations to which it belongs, and the same may be said of an instant. In referring to the complexity of terms within terms Spaulding says, "Ultimately, . . . there must be simple terms that make all this complexity possible, but that are themselves not complex. . . . Points and instants are examples of such ultimate simple terms."[18] He may be wrong in further maintaining

[17] Russell, *The Principles of Mathematics*, p. 212.
[18] Spaulding, *The New Rationalism*, p. 178.

that these simple terms are independent, but he holds that they are at least implied by the complexities of terms within terms, that is, by the relations in which they stand. And indeed there seems to be no reason for assuming that these simple terms subsist independently. Terms and relations, so far as present knowledge goes, may imply ultimate simple terms but they do not imply that such simple terms are independent of the relations which imply them. This conception of ultimate simple terms may be called the theory of the internality of ultimate terms. Most terms then turn out to be relations or systems of relations. Even such terms as "sensations," or "bits of matter," which might at first seem to be ultimate terms may turn out to be relations. And if certain terms like "points" and "instants" cannot themselves be reduced to relations they are implied by the system of relations in which they stand, by space and by time. Truth instead of being a system of terms and relations seems to have become a system of relations with a few questionable terms which are secondary to the relations.

The criticism of this second view of relation as the foundation to the theory of truth leads to the following results: First, all relations must be relating relations, otherwise they would not perform their proper function of relating and would tend to become terms in the analytical relation; secondly, terms must be either relations or factors standing in relation, otherwise they would be isolated entities and have no place in the system of truth; and thirdly, relations rather than terms are dominant in the system of truth. This second view, that truth is made up of terms and relations, is unsatisfactory because in fact the relations seem to crowd out the terms. This emphasis on relation fits in well with the coherence theory of truth, but it also suggests the third view of relation.

The theory of truth as based upon the third view of relation may be called the relational theory of truth. According to this theory, the center of gravity lies in the relations. The terminal theory emphasizes the terms and does not work out the full character of relation. The terminal-relational theory cannot maintain its balance; it either tends to treat all terms and relations as terms in the analytical relation and therefore becomes primarily a terminal theory, or it gives full scope to relations as relating relations, thereby pushing the terms into the background, and so leads on to the relational theory. The relational theory, however, is not misled by making any concessions to terms; it makes relations in their full meaning fundamental to truth. Fixed groups of relations, such as things which may be terms in further relations, are recognized as essentially relations, and the specific character of relation is not mistaken for its full character. This theory thus makes truth a system of relations of relations and allows of ultimate terms only as terminals of relations and as implied by relations.

If, then, terms are relations or implications of relations and truth is a system of relations, why should terms be considered at all as having an important place in the system of truth? It might be thought that while terms have figured in the earlier theories of truth they are of little value in the relational theory which makes relations fundamental. To answer that according to the relational theory relations imply terms would be unsatisfactory because the terms are themselves relations and instead of saying that relations imply terms it could be said that relations imply further relations. The real reason why the conception of term is retained in a relational theory of truth is to be found primarily in the nature of relation. A relation as essentially a relating relation implies something related to something; the somethings are the terminals of the relation, the manifold brought to unity in the relation. Terms are the terminals of relations though they themselves may be relational in character. There is a further reason for retaining the conception of term. A term as a terminal of a relation not only may be terminal to the relation, but may be itself highly complex. The planet Venus as terminal to many relations in the solar system is itself a very elaborate system or whole of relations; a triangle as a terminal in a relation of congruity to another triangle is in its own nature very complex. But the complexity of a terminal, though it may be in some measure relevant to the relation in which it stands, is not needed in expressing that relation. The proposition *Venus receives heat from the sun,* as expressing a relation of Venus to the sun, is not concerned with the complexity of Venus but treats it as a whole; nor is a triangle treated other than as a whole when it is said to be congruent to another triangle. And not only is a proposition expressing the relation of terms not concerned with the intricacies of the terms, but it is primarily the expression of a relation of the terms as wholes or units. Since, then, it is essential to the structure of truth to regard the terminals of relations as units or as wholes, the conception of term is of value in characterizing systems or wholes of relations as terminals of further relations.

Relations imply terminals, and terms are the terminals of relations. That terms are not called merely relations related, relations standing in further relations, is due to the further character of most but not all terms that they are systems of relations complex in themselves and capable of being terminals to more than one relation. They are like beads on a chain, often being fixed in character and retaining their fixed character when their relations to one another are changed, as when beads are strung upon a new string. But this further character is not found in all terms; some of them seem to be simple. Points and instants reveal no inner complexity. Therefore, they are terms merely as terminals to the relations in the relational system in which they stand. A number system, which is more general than space or time, reveals in its terms, the numbers, the same characteristic. A number is an empty term in an order. Unlike a bead on a chain or a brick in a building, it contains no complexity but is simply terminal to the order or system of relations making up the number system. It conforms to the primary conception of a term as a terminal, but is not a relation or a whole of relations. It is a bare unit in a system which implies it. Unlike number, a sensation seems to have a character over and above the relations in which it stands. The quality blue in perception might well be red instead without any real difference in its relations being involved. If so, the relations in which a sensation stands would not determine the character of the sensation, yet the quality of sensation seems to be simple and to involve no complexity. But, as was said above, the sensation may be complex and still not be analyzable by the mind. Sensation, therefore, suggests nothing further with respect to the nature of terms. Terms, then, in the system of truth are actually relations, or groups of relations taken as wholes, or ultimate factors implied by relations; as relevant to relations they are the terminals of relations, either simple ultimate terminals or terminals involving further complexity.

If most terms turn out to be relations, then certainly it may be said that many relations are also terms; and if it be further recognized that all relations may be regarded as possible terms, it may be asked why truth may not be said to consist of a system of terms rather than of a system of relations. The world might be said to be made up of terms within terms, or of highly complex groups of terms. Such a system of truth would be like a collection of entities finding its unity in the group. Truth might be conceived in this way, but such a conception of it would be very inadequate. Either it would be a bare collection or it would stand in need of the conception of relation to give essential character to most of its terms. As a bare collection its unity would lie only in the unity of the group and the specific connections among the terms would not play the part of actually relating; and if the relating function of the terms is recognized, then it becomes a question as to whether term or relation expresses the more fundamental nature of truth. It would seem in a coherence theory of truth that relation rather than term would constitute the most essential character of truth as a synthetic system. Truth as synthetic is primarily relation or a system of relations. Terms are the terminals of relations, and if they reveal inner complexity that complexity is essentially relational. However valuable the conception of terms may be, it is secondary to the conception of relation.

In the relational theory of truth it is important to note that, as all relations are relating relations, the unity of the relation cannot be separated from its specific character: not of course that the unity and the specific character are not distinguishable, but that both are essential to relation. The unity is a formal character of the relation and is not something which is added by the proposition. In the example *a causes b, cause* not only has specific character as cause but has the character of relating *b* with *a*. It is not as if there were an *a*, a specific character *cause*, and *b*, and that then the proposition united them. The unity springs from the relation and not from the proposition. The proposition is nothing more than a relation, or the expression of a relation, provided the relation is understood to mean a relating relation and implies its terms so far as they are terminal to it. All that belongs to the relation may be expressed in the proposition, but all that is found in the proposition must be grounded in the relation. If it be said that a proposition as distinguished from a relation is an assertion, it may be answered that this only means that the proposition holds in a larger body of truth; but as truth is a system of relations there must be ground for the assertion in the nexus of relations to which the relation expressed in the proposition belongs. In other words, propositions even as assertions are grounded in relation or relational systems, and the relations not only supply variety of connection in the relational system but actually connect and unify it.

Beside unity and specific character, relation includes direction. As Russell says, "it is characteristic of a relation of two terms that it proceeds, so to speak, from one to the other." Of the two propositions " 'A is greater than B' and 'B is greater than A,' " he says, "These two propositions, though different, contain precisely the same constituents." [19] It would be impossible to express the difference between these two propositions on the basis of the terminals *A* and *B* or of the specific character of the relation; and even the unity of the relation would not be sufficient to bring out the difference if the unity were not a uniting in one direction or the other, a connecting *A* with *B* or *B* with *A*. This factor of direction in relation is important in two ways. On the one hand it suggests that relation is not a mere static grouping of terms but involves a from–to character and thus gives foundation to transi-

[19] Russell, *The Principles of Mathematics*, pp. 95, 107.

tion and movement. A grouping of terms, however well unified, would not, without the factor of direction, contain any ground leading to connection with other relations. The nexus of relations forming truth would then not be a genuinely interrelated system. That *A is greater than B* suggests that *B may be greater than C*. The transition from *A* to *B* continues on from *B* to *C*. This fitting of the direction of one relation to the direction of another through their common terminal is the basis of number, order, continuity, systematic implication, and the general interrelation of relations, and is grounded in this factor of direction in relation. On the other hand, direction affects and complicates the unity in multiple relation. In the commonly used example *a gives m to b* the relation has more than two terms. Where does direction come in? It can hardly be a sort of general direction among the terms. Just as the terms are many, so the directions are many; there would seem to be as many directions as there are terms which can be paired. There is direction from *a* to *m*, from the giver to the gift; there is direction from *m* to *b*, from the gift to the receiver; there is direction from *a* to *b*, the giver to the receiver; and there is also direction from *a* to *bRm*, the giver to *b* as receiver of the gift, and again of *aRb* to *m* and of *aRm* to *b*. A multiple relation seems to be a group of two-term relations each having its direction, and there would seem to be further relations between the group as a whole and the particular relations. A multiple relation may be a more or less complicated system of relations involving some kind of grouping, but whether it is called a multiple relation or a system of relations the factor of direction as well as the multiplicity of terms adds to its complexity. Thus direction plays a vital part in the relational system of truth.

Relation implies terms, and the factor of direction adds to the force of this implication. Furthermore, the terms may be more or less complex. But now it may be asked how relation is connected with its terms. Does the connection involve any further complication? and does the character of the terms determine the relation? or does the character of the relation determine the terms? Bradley says if a relation is to "be something" to its terms then "a new connecting relation" will be required, and this new relation will then require further connecting relations to connect it with the original relation and the terms. This procedure will then lead on to an infinite regress of connecting relations, a "hopeless process, since we are forced to go on finding new relations without end." [20] To say that such further relations are implied by a relation and that they relate this relation to its terms may be true, but this original relation does not need these further relations to do its relating. A relation relating its terms is original and not reducible to any further relations. Though it be granted that the relation is directly connected with its terms, it may still be maintained that the specific character of the relation may or must affect the character of the terms and that the specific character of the terms may or must affect the character of the relation. Much has been said in recent years about the "internality" and "externality" of relations. According to the internal theory, the character of a relation is grounded in the character of its terms, and it might conversely be said that the character of relation implies a specific character in its terms. According to the external theory, the specific character of relations and terms do not imply each other necessarily. Terms may imply relations and relations may imply terms, but so far as the formal character of relation goes, terms and relations are independent. The first theory makes for complete implication between terms and their relations in the whole field of truth, and the second theory, while admitting that implication is possible in some relations, does not make implication essential to all relations. The relational theory of truth as accepted in this work cannot accept the internal theory. Complete implication is not grounded in fact, the internal theory is extreme and unwarranted and has no basis in the formal nature of relation. The external theory is on the whole acceptable. So far as the essential nature of relation goes, relations may be of both kinds, internal and external.

[20] Francis Herbert Bradley, *Appearance and Reality* (2nd ed., London, 1897), pp. 32–33.

Whether relations are internal or external cannot be determined by the form but only by the matter of the relations. There might seem to be an exception in the case of such terms as numbers, points, and instants. The theory of the internality of ultimate terms, as explained above, holds that such ultimate simple terms are determined by the relations in which they stand. While the formal character of relation implies such terms as terminals, it is only the material character of the relations in which they stand which determines the character of these terms. The formal character of relation for the relational theory of truth must then be original and not be referred to further relations, and it must be free and neutral with respect to material implication. Though truth without any material implication would be a hopeless chaos, so far as it is based upon the formal character of relation it must leave room for all possible kinds of relations.

Enough has been said to bring out the general character of the relational theory of truth and to show how it centers in the conception of relation. It was pointed out that the terminal theory was inadequate because it made relations attributes of terms or things and did not do justice to their full character. This was historically the earliest theory, but owing to its neglect of the real importance of relation it led to another theory, the terminal-relational theory. According to this second theory, truth was said to consist of relations as well as terms so that the fundamental place of relations along with terms was recognized. This is the theory most commonly held today, but the foregoing criticism has shown it to be unstable. It either led to the treatment of relations as too independent or as terms in the analytical relation, or it led to the recognition that most terms were relations and thus made relations more fundamental than terms. It was then shown that this theory naturally led to the consideration of relations as central to the theory of truth, and the theory of truth making relations central was called the relational theory of truth. This theory should now be recognized as a theory standing out in contrast with the other two theories. It makes relations fundamental, original, and central. Terms are not independent of and over and above relations; they are essentially terminals of relations; they are involved in the nature of relation as relating relations. If these terminals are complex they turn out to be relations or groups of relations, and if they are simple ultimate terminals they are merely implications of relations in which they stand. All comes back to relation and all systems of truth are grounded in relation.

Furthermore, the formal nature of relation as the foundation of the relational theory of truth has been defined as a unity involving specific character, terminals, and direction. Relation so defined is the unit of truth, and through its essentially connected character it forms the basis of a nexus of relations, a system of interrelations of relations. This definition of the formal side of relation leaves the material side undetermined. That a relation has specific character, terms, and direction is a formal matter; but the type or particular nature of its specific character, terms, and direction is material. So far as the definition goes, the relation on its material side might be as loose as the relation "and," or it might express implication between its terms, as is largely the case in mathematics. Should it be said that because relation implies terms the definition implies the internality of terms, it may be pointed out that this would only hold of the definition as formal, but that inasmuch as the material side of relation is left undetermined by the definition, the external theory would hold for the material of the relation. The definition suggests only the general character of relation as the form of truth, and leaves the detail and more special character of the relations making up truth undetermined.

The definition and significance of relation as the foundation of truth was developed in order to make explicit the fundamental note in the coherence theory — its connective, synthetic, or relational character. The conception of the "significant whole" and the conception of the mutual implication of the contents usually included in this theory being disregarded, it may be said that the synthetic or connective principle as worked out in the relational theory supplies a beginning to the positive structure of truth. The correspondence theory was rejected in favor of the coherence theory because this latter theory seems to have more to suggest with regard to the positive structure. But it was noted that the factor of error was better accounted for by the correspondence theory. To account for the factor of error some modification or enlargement of the structure of truth may be necessary, as will be shown later. The intuitional theory may also have something to suggest as to the determination of truth, though it has nothing to offer with regard to its positive structure. Before account is taken of the suggestions coming from the correspondence and intuitional theories more must be said with regard to the positive structure of truth, some evidence must be presented to show that it is grounded in coherence and relation.

To show that relation is fundamental to truth means, on the one hand, to show that all truths are essentially relational or based on relation, and, on the other hand, to show that relation is not reducible to anything else, to anything nonrelational. To make clear that all truths are relational or based on relation it should be noted that any truth which can be adduced or imagined or thought of will reveal itself in relational form. The expression of truth in propositions is always relational, and if a proposition includes certain ultimate terms which are not relations it need only be remembered that such terms can be shown to be essentially terminals of relations and therefore based on relation. Should it be thought that possibly some truth may appear which will turn out not to be relational or based upon relation, then it should be noted further that if anything is true it has character, that is, it has quality, and as qualitative it is either identical with or different from other things. Now as identical or different it stands in relation, and if its character is complex the factors making up its character will be as to their quality either identical with or different from each other, its character thus showing itself to be relational. A thing, then, whether considered with respect to itself or with respect to other things, is, so far as it has quality, relational; and the same might be said with respect to its quantity. It is only necessary to ask whether truth, if it has any meaning at all, can escape being relation. The answer depends upon analysis, and the above analysis has shown that relation is inescapable, that meaning or character is relational in form. As a result any item of truth would either be relation or stand in relation. Analysis then reveals the omnipresence of relation, thus proving that all truth is relational.

Though the content of all truth is relation, relation might be reducible to some other form. Therefore relation must be shown to be original and irreducible. If it should be held that relation is not original, but reducible, because its specific character of relation and its terms must be related through a further relation or because the unity, specific character, direction, and terms of a relation must be referred to the analytical relation of difference, such arguments will be of no avail; for relation is not then reduced to something other than relation but only to further relation, and relation is thus not escaped. But if the fact is neglected that the four formal characters of relation are revealed through analysis it might be claimed that these characters are distinct entities or beings, and that relation is made up of these entities and is therefore reducible to them. It might even be said that the character of unity actually unifies or connects the terms while still retaining its own being, and that the terms play the part of terminals in relation though they retain their own being. It is unimportant whether the view here maintained is to be identified with the terminal-relational theory of truth — that truth consists of terms and relations — or whether it is just a question of the factors of relation revealed by analysis. The view assumes that relation is based on entities or beings which are more fundamental. In answer to the contention that entity or being is more fundamental than relation, it may be said that if the unity of the relation unites the terms this unity is more significant as relating than as being or entity. To treat it as an entity is an attempt to treat it as a kind of term which is not terminal to any relation; but terms have meaning either as terminals of relations or as relations themselves, and, in so far as ultimate terms go, there is no evidence that there are any which are not essentially terminals. But it may still be maintained that entity or being is more fundamental than relation. It may be said that being is more fundamental because it is more universal. It will be argued either that the four formal characters of relation as four different kinds need a more fundamental conception under which they may be grouped, or that terms are distinct from relations and therefore there must be a more fundamental category of being to include them both. The answer is: the four formal characters of relation, since they are phases of relation, should be classed as relation; and terms, since they are relations or factors in relation, need not be classed separately from relation; therefore, since there is nothing beside relation, relation is as universal as being. If a being cannot stand by itself, and if as a factor in relation it expresses its essential character, then relation would seem to be more original than being and not reducible to it; and if being is no more universal than relation in range, then it cannot be regarded as a more general concept to which relation can be reduced.

Another argument for the originality of relation is possible. Relation, it says, is connection or synthesis, and synthesis is original. A synthesis may be broken up by analysis, but always with a view to making a fuller and better synthesis. The procedure in philosophy and science is from synthesis to analysis and then on to synthesis again, the analysis revealing factors which make a deeper and more accurate synthesis possible. The beginning and end of all methods would seem to be synthesis. Relation as synthesis may be analyzed, but the factors which the analysis distinguishes are of use only in making clearer the full meaning of relation as synthesis. If a relation is broken up into its component parts it is no longer a relation, but if it is regarded as a relation or synthesis which includes in its nature certain distinguishable factors it is still a relation, and as a relation it is primary. The unit of synthesis is relation, full relating relation involving terminals. If truth is essentially synthesis then its units cannot be reduced to anything less than relation. The core or form of relation cannot be disrupted, it is original and irreducible.

The proof of the coherence theory, the proof that relation is fundamental, has been worked out by showing that all truths are essentially relational and that relation is irreducible. It might, of course, be said that even if relation is not reducible to being, it is itself being, and therefore the conception of being might be regarded as fundamental. No doubt, the conception of being could then be substituted for the conception of relation, but as it would mean the same as relation nothing essential would be accomplished. Of the two terms, relation and being, relation would seem to be preferable because it is more suggestive of the character of truth, while being is empty and connotes little. Though being is not more fundamental than relation, it might still be held that being is more fundamental than truth — that truth as a whole is a phase of a world of being and only expressive of one aspect of being. If there is the least hint that being is a reality or an existence and that truth is an attribute of it, then most certainly truth is the fuller and more complete conception because reality and existence express that which actually is, whereas truth covers all possible relations, all that is possible. To say that something is or has being, or has character at all, is to say that it is relational and therefore belongs to truth. As relational, being is a function of truth, since truth is the all-inclusive conception.

This relational theory of truth leads to a kind of logical idealism or formal idealism. It is not concerned with the relation of truth to a subject or mind, it merely expresses a synthetic or relational conception of the world of truth rather than a more realistic conception of the world as made up of independent entities, or terms and relations, or separate bits of existence. It stands for the connective rather than the separative view of things. The formal nature of relation is the beginning of the central core of truth on which the great syntheses and organized conceptions of science and philosophy are based, whereas the analysis of the world into entities or terms and relations leads only to the differentiation of the various types of entities but not to any consideration of the nature of relation to the syntheses of knowledge. The method of realism is analytic, that of logical idealism synthetic. The reference to idealism is here merely suggested; its real significance will be more apparent after the further account has been given of the structure and arrangement of the content of truth.

Up to this point truth has been considered as a system or nexus of relations, the relations having a certain formal nature. Nothing was said about its content or matter over and above its formal character except possibly that ultimate terms are implied by the relations in which they stand, as explained in the theory of internality of ultimate terms. The formal character of relation, both in making relations specific and in implying terms, points to contents which are definite; but while it involves contents, it leaves room for all possible kinds of relations as contents. Truth must have the form of relation; it must consist of relating relations; but the relations may be of infinite variety. These relations need not imply each other; they may be loose or compact as long as they are connected and form a nexus.

But now it may be pointed out that certain relations can be found in the world of truth which involve implication, and it may then be asked whether the fact is of any significance to the structure of truth. Are such relations involving implication merely incidental, that is, only unimportant parts of the nexus of truth not contributing anything essential to its structure? or are these relations vital to the interconnection of relations and essential to the structure of truth? The question may be made more specific. If there is implication between one relation and another, or between one group of relations and another, then one relation is the condition of the other or one group of relations is the condition of the other group, and it may be asked whether the condition may not condition many other relations or groups and therefore serve as a principle or determining relation or some phase or part of the system of relations or indeed of the whole system. In the postulates of a geometrical system, in the causal law of nature, or in a moral principle, such determining relations are to be found. In other words, is truth as a system of relations like an intricate net with some parts more closely woven than other parts but with no part determining all the other parts, or is it like a building, part of which, the foundation, conditions and defines the general shape of the rest of the building?

As far as the formal nature of relation goes it might seem as if the structure of truth as a nexus of relations could be like a net, but the following considerations make clear that it has rather the character of a building. In the first place, truth is synthetic; its contents must conform to the character of relation and it is an intricate mass of relations, relations of relations of relations. As synthetic and as intricate it must contain not only elaborate relations or complex groups of relations but also relations relating major parts of the system and including them as terms; and if it be noted that every part of the system must stand in some relation not necessarily in implicated relation to every other part, then some relations or groups of relations will be highly inclusive if not all-inclusive. Such inclusive relations limit and thus condition other relations and so become their foundation. This massing of relations due to the full play of their synthetic character is of the highest importance and suggests that the structure of truth includes fundamental relations.

Then a consideration of types of relation points toward a foundation. There being likenesses in the field of truth, there are therefore types of relation. A type is a universal or universal relation, and a universal relation has a twofold character. On the one hand it expresses a specific relational character as distinct from other relations, and on the other hand it defines, refers to, or includes under itself, particulars — that is, through its character it defines the character of certain particular relations or groups of relations which are otherwise differentiated. One type of universal may be included within another more general type of universal and that again within another which is still more general. The most general universals would then limit all less general universals so that just as any universal defines particulars the most general universals define the whole system, unifying and limiting it and so becoming fundamental to it. Identity, difference, unity, order, implication, and causality are examples of relations with high degree of universality.

Furthermore, relations of a high degree of universality seem to be actually implied or presupposed in any system of truth. Such relations are said to be the necessary conditions of the system. The postulates of a geometrical system condition the whole system. The physical world implies order as a necessary condition. All systems of truth imply identity, difference, multiplicity, and the primary conditions of number. Not only, then, are there universals which are conditions, but also there are universals which are necessary conditions. The necessary universals form a body of fundamental relations, a *sine qua non*, of all systems of truth. The synthetic character of relation, the types of relation, and implication in relational systems, all point in the direction of such a *sine qua non*, a fundamental core of truth.

This nucleus of necessary universals may be called the logical core; and it would seem that there are two methods by which the mind can make it evident that there is such a core: first, by raising the question as to how synthesis is carried out, how relation relates, and by showing that as relation actually relates it relates definitely and so connects by means of specific character or quality, and that as it relates terms and exhibits direction it connects by uniting a plurality of factors, that is, through quantity; and secondly, by starting with any relation in the system of truth, then working back by reduction to the most general principles presupposed by it, and finding these principles in the syntheses or relations of quality and quantity. Both methods reveal both qualitative and quantitative relations in the core. The relations of quality are identity and difference. It would be impossible to conceive of any system of truth without these two fundamental relations. The factors in a system in order to have any meaning at all would have to be definitely something, and these factors, in so far as they have the same character, are qualitatively identical, and in so far as they have varying character are qualitatively different. Once qualities are given, identity and difference cannot be escaped; and these two qualitative relations are the basis of universals, classes, and groups. The relations of quantity are unity and plurality. If there are any relations at all there will be unity and plurality. The full meaning of these two quantitative relations involves number, including order. The fundamental or universal relations of identity, difference, unity, plurality, and number would seem to be necessary to all systems of truth — that is, if there is a system of relations at all, these universals are implied.

Though these universals form a sort of central core to truth, it should be noted that any special system of truth may also have its own special core. The special core of a mathematical system is to be found in its postulates, which define and condition the whole system. The special core of a moral system is to be found in the presuppositions which condition the moral laws or moral order of purposes and ends. In the same way the physical world is specifically conditioned by the presuppositions of the quantitative structure of space and time and of the order of events in space and time as expressed in the causal relation. If to the necessary universal relations forming the central core are added the universal relations necessary to the special systems of truth, the logical core becomes fuller and richer and includes all fundamental necessary relations as first principles of truth. This full logical core might be said to be made up of postulates, of all the postulates of truth. But as the term postulate suggests something rather arbitrarily chosen it is not the best term to use particularly with reference to the central core which is necessary to all truth. Fundamental presuppositions or necessary conditions would better suggest the character of the universal relations included in the core.

The significance of these universal relations and their function in the system of truth cannot be overestimated. Their value to knowledge has been fully recognized since the days of Socrates and Plato. They are peculiarly significant relations, and without them the human mind could not attain to any genuine knowledge. Aristotle in his table of categories tried to define the most fundamental of these relations, but in Kant there is to be found a truly systematic account of them. Kant's system of categories with their deduction offers the first appreciation of the fundamental synthetic function of these relations as principles of truth. Cohen,[21] Natorp,[22] and Cassirer [23] have developed Kant's thought more fully and adjusted it to the more recent developments in philosophy.

The logical core consists, then, of the fundamental necessary conditions of all truth, including not only its indispensable conditions but also the more special conditions which form the essential relations of the various branches of truth. These conditions are the basis of truth as an ordered system. Every truth implies the core and therefore is a function of it. Because of the core it has its place in the order. If the logical core defines and conditions all truth, then infinite truth is dependent on it and conditioned by it. In other words, truth being infinite, the core forms the foundation to a structure of infinite proportions.

As truth is an infinite nexus of relations and yet is centered in certain fundamental relations it may be said to have a beginning but no end. Logic, as the science of the core, as the science of these fundamental relations, is the science of beginnings; all other sciences and branches of knowledge are concerned with the infinite ramifications of truth beyond the core. It may be objected that this centering of truth in the core is an arranging of relations in a scale based upon their universality, and that however useful this arrangement may be for the systematizing of knowledge it is essentially arbitrary; or if not arbitrary, at least of no vital importance to the structure of truth. But it should be remembered that the universal relations of the core are not only universal but necessary and implied as the condition *sine qua non* of the relations beyond the core. Any relation or group of relations beyond the core may be said to imply and presuppose the core; the truth of any science implies the truth of logic. The

[21] Hermann Cohen, *Logik der reinen Erkenntniss* (Berlin, 1902).

[22] Paul Natorp, *Die logischen Grundlagen der exakten Wissenschaften* (2nd ed., Leipzig and Berlin, 1921).

[23] Ernst Cassirer, *Substanzbegriff und Funktionsbegriff* (Berlin, 1910).

necessity of implication of universal relations, not their universality, is the essential basis of the conception of the core. To overlook the necessary relations of the core is to neglect something which conditions and therefore permeates or cuts down through all truth; it is to neglect not only a vital feature of truth but also that which gives to it order and organization. The conception of the core suggests, then, a unity and order inwrought in the structure of truth.

The foregoing development of the conception of the logical core makes it clear that truth consists neither of independent entities, nor of a bare network of relations, nor of groups of relations based on arbitrarily chosen postulates, but rather of a system of relations based on a nucleus of certain necessary relations or conditions, the nucleus being the foundation of an ordered system. Truth is thus a function of its core. This fundamentally synthetic view is quite clearly a form of logical or formal idealism, and it expresses this idealism in a more profound way than was suggested above in connection with the formal character of truth. If idealism means a philosophy of form, a theory that everything is a function of certain fundamental forms in contrast with the realistic theory of independent entities, then the conception of truth as centered in the core is clearly an idealistic theory. The relational theory of truth, by making truth consist of relations — that is, by making it a function of relational form — is idealistic in outline; but the full synthetic or connective theory of truth as a function of the core excludes any possibility of a realistic conception of separate entities by regarding form not only as relational form but as something central and fundamental in the system of truth.

This connective, as opposed to the separative, view of truth so far as it is relational in form does not, as was said above, involve the internality of relations. The content of truth may include internal or external relations, implicative or non-implicative relations. But it may now be asked whether the conception of the core does not make all truth implicative and therefore make all content conform to the theory of internality. The answer is simple. To the extent to which any specific truth or relation presupposes the logical core, so far implication is essential, otherwise not. The content of truth must conform to the core, but so far as its details go the core may not determine it. That which is in space must conform to the quantitative character of space, but its further character, its specific configuration in space, is not determined by quantitative relation. So far as space goes the particular configuration of an object in one part of space may be quite external to that of an object in another part of space. A moral principle may determine the correct form of a great variety of acts, but the greater part of the detail of these acts may not be determined by the moral principle. The core is not the whole of truth. It conditions all truth but does not determine all the phases and the detail of its content. Once more the analogy of the building will make this clear. The foundation is necessary, and implied by the rest of the building; above the foundation, however, the building may be constructed in many and various ways. Both necessity and contingency have their place in truth. One relation may imply the core yet not imply every other relation. Implication may have originally suggested the core, but the core has turned out to be only a logical beginning, a fundamental form, not an exhaustive necessity.

The consideration of the structure of truth has led to two important results: truth is relational and truth is a function of the core. That truth is relational in form, that it is a system of relations, was suggested by the coherence theory. That truth is a function of the core, that it presupposes certain fundamental relations, was arrived at by taking account of the implications and interrelations of the relations in the system of truth, that is, by taking account of the content of truth. As relational and as implying the core, truth has a definite structure. But as was pointed out earlier in this chapter, some place must be found in the theory of truth for error. The correspondence theory was found unsatisfactory except on the negative side, that is, it was accepted only in so far as it recognized error as an essential feature in the structure of truth. The theory of truth as a system of relations, no matter how well grounded in a core, might seem to suggest a positive definite structure, a very elaborate structure, but by its very character of definiteness allowing no place for indefiniteness, ambiguity, or error. How then can a place be found for error in the structure of truth?

It is natural to think of error as involving an erring mind, but to regard truth in itself as beyond error. To say that the mind might have ideas of its own and that these ideas might be different from the truth which they were intended to represent is only to revert to the dualistic difficulties of the correspondence theory. Suppose, however, mind were to face truth directly, to be immediately conscious of truth, then error could not be explained through the relation of mind to truth. It would be possible then to find a place for error only in the structure of truth. The definiteness of truth might seem to exclude error from its structure, but it should be remembered that its definiteness is not complete. If truth is taken as a nexus of relations it may be said of it that any relation or any group of relations however extensive leaves further relations untouched. Truth is not only definite but it is also inexhaustible and therefore indefinite. This indefiniteness makes error possible. The infinite manifoldness of relations makes it impossible for any definite set of relations to define truth without leaving an undefined residuum. With respect to that which is defined the residuum may be what it may — the undefined, the indefinite, the region of error.

But now it may be objected that truth as a system of relations is definite *ad infinitum,* that is, that it is made up of an unlimited number of definite relations, and that as all of its relations are definite there is no room for indefiniteness. Though every relation, it may be answered, is definite in itself, no single relation or finite group of relations can fully define or condition all of the other relations, so that relative to any finite set of relations other relations are indefinite. Take for example the sun. No matter what relations are used by the astronomers to define or designate it, those relations do not condition it in all its concreteness nor do they necessitate all the detail of further relations which are needed fully to define it. Or consider truth as grounded in the core. The core includes certain fundamental and necessary relations, and these relations define the whole field of truth in certain fundamental ways, but they are quite ambiguous with respect to the special relations of the particular systems of truth. The relations composing truth may be arranged in order of universality beginning with the fundamental relations of the core, but there is no fundamental relation or principle stretching out from the core which can determine the whole series of relations. In mechanics a formula may be given defining the variable velocity of a moving point moving toward a limit, and this formula may define the velocity at every point through which the moving point passes. The formula thus covers the velocities at all the points, the number of such points being infinite. Now there is no formula or fundamental relation like the mechanical formula which can define all the relations in a system of truth. All the relations may be definite, but there is no gathering them up under one relation or one group of relations. The most universal relation may penetrate but never exhaust all other relations. Thus indefiniteness is involved in the interrelatedness of relations.

But why, it may still be objected, must truth be conceived as grouped under a finite set of relations? It may be a fact that a finite set of relations is only part of truth and that this part is indefinite with respect to further parts, but why is this indefiniteness significant? All truth as truth is definite. The mind in its search for truth knows only part of the truth and therefore is indefinite with regard to the rest, but this does not affect truth itself. The mind may strive to grasp truth under a limited number of universal relations, but because the mind cannot exhaust truth in this way it should not be said that the resulting indefiniteness is due to the nature of truth when it is really due to the relation of the mind to truth. In answer to this further objection it should be conceded that a particular case of indefiniteness does involve a mind, but at the same time it should be pointed out that the ground of indefiniteness is contained in the structure of truth. Only a mind in its incomplete grasp of truth can actually err, but the fact that the part of truth which the mind grasps cannot as a phase of truth define all truth is a fact due to truth and not to the mind.

And not only is the possibility of indefiniteness bound up with the structure of truth but most of the relations composing truth actually suggest further relations without fully defining them: aRb suggests bRc, but the specific character of the first R does not necessarily suggest the specific character of the second R. Time implies events without fully defining them, as also a moral law implies moral acts. Thus the synthetic structure of truth in this very positive way includes a kind of indefiniteness. If the relations composing truth were so tightly bound together that one relation implied all other relations, then there would be no room for indefiniteness and error. But truth shows no such compactness. As synthetic, its relations are connected and grouped, they are the function of a core; but since its relations are not all implicative the possibility of indefiniteness and error is grounded in truth.

Should it be maintained that indefiniteness is not error, that it is at most a kind of ambiguity but not positive error, it may be pointed out that though indefiniteness is not error in the sense of being a definite mistake or false suggestion, it does make error possible and is the logical foundation of error in the structure of truth. If truth were constructed differently, if the relations composing it were absolutely compact, then the possibility of error could not be found in the structure of truth. The mind may make mistakes and thus err with respect to truth whatever its nature, but error in scientific hypotheses is not primarily mental, it can be explained only by reference to the indefiniteness involved in the composition of truth. Error, then, is the result of indefiniteness.

Factors suggested by the coherence and correspondence theories of truth have now been shown to be involved in the structure of truth, and an outline of this structure has been presented. Its structure has been shown to involve a definite form and content with a resulting indefiniteness on which error is based. The logical core gives unity to the structure, but a unity which does not interfere with the infinite variety of the relations composing it. Truth is, then, a vast system of relations centered in a core.

If to be true means to be relational or to be a relation in a system of relations centering in a core, then being true would not seem to involve being known. But the importance of being known, of the relation of the mind to truth, is brought out by the intuitional theory. This theory suggests nothing as to the structure of truth, but it does suggest something as to the point of view from which truth must be considered. According to this theory there must be an intuition of truth, a direct relation of the mind to truth if truth is to be known, though the intuition must in no way affect truth. As Descartes says, the mind should start with the apprehension of a simple truth or proposition and then move on to the apprehension of more complex truths; that is, it should see clearly and distinctly the truth with which it starts as also each further truth to which it proceeds. No doubt Descartes thought that the truths apprehended by this procedure were connected by some sort of implication, but so far as his view suggests connection and implication it is concerned with the structure of truth and is therefore no proper part of the intuitional theory but rather a phase of the coherence theory. A clear and distinct apprehension or intuition of the truth is the essential feature of the intuitional theory. To see truth clearly the mind must plunge in and swim. In other words, to know truth the mind must first start with some relation, proposition, or truth, and then move on to further relations, propositions, or truths without limit. As truth is infinite and inexhaustible and the human mind is finite and limited it is not possible for the mind to know all truth in one intuition. Therefore, knowledge can be attained only gradually, step by step. Since this procedure is necessary for knowledge, necessary in order that there be any science or philosophy at all, the question as to the access to truth as well as the question as to its structure must be considered in any thoroughgoing account of truth.

How then is the access to truth related to the structure of truth? or how is knowledge related to truth? If truth is primary and knowledge of it secondary, knowledge is a kind of identification or contact of the mind with truth. As such, knowledge is limited; it never includes all truth. If the whole truth were the only true truth, then knowledge of the truth would be impossible, but this assumption need not be made, as was pointed out in considering the coherence theory. Knowledge as limited is knowledge of a part only of the structure of truth, but the part known may be considered to be true as a part. Whatever is known may be so far true. Knowledge may start with any part of truth, with any relation or group of relations, and must start with some relation or group. This relation or group of relations forms a nucleus to which further relations are added, and the nucleus with these added relations then forms a larger nucleus to which still further relations may be added. A body of knowledge is thus formed as a basis for further expansion. In this way truth is appropriated more and more by knowledge, and knowledge identifies itself more and more with the system of relations composing truth.

Knowledge being a gradual and expanding identification of the mind with inexhaustible truth, it is at any stage in the process limited, but at the same time unlimited with respect to its possible progress and expansion. Any relation may serve as a starting point and any body of truth may represent a stage in the progress of knowledge, but it is more common to think of the body of positive knowledge as developed by science and philosophy as a starting point or stage in knowledge upon which further knowledge and research is to be built. In other words, positive knowledge is a base or nucleus of determined knowledge with respect to which further knowledge is to be determined. It may be convenient to speak of the body of positive or determined knowledge as the *abc* of knowledge, and to call that which is to be determined and is not yet determined the *x* of knowledge. The *abc* of knowledge may also be called the epistemological core. If to be true is to be relational, then to be known is to be determined. To be determined means to be definitely included in the *abc* of knowledge. The progress of knowledge then means that the *x* gradually becomes part of the *abc*, or it may be said that the *abc* eats into the *x* — the epistemological core grows at the expense of the *x*. But now it should be noted that, since knowledge is a process, truth as known must be considered from the point of view of knowledge, which is dynamic and moving. There is no direct way to complete an absolute truth. Truth can be conceived only relative to knowledge, and since knowledge is dynamic, involving the *abc–x* process, the perspective of truth may be affected by knowledge.

In the consideration of the relation of knowledge to truth two questions very naturally arise. First, why is this relation of any great significance? As long as it is recognized that knowledge does not affect the structure of truth and that the known truth is only a part of truth and therefore not to be mixed up with the truth which is not yet known, the problem of knowledge ought to cause no difficulty. Once see clearly that knowledge is of a finite amount of truth, to which, to be sure, additions can be made, keep within the bounds of knowledge and do not lay claim to knowledge of truth which is not yet known, and the relation of knowledge to truth becomes very simple. Secondly, why are there not as many epistemological cores as there are minds seeking truth? Or, if it be realized that the knowledge of an individual mind is part of the general body of positive knowledge, why are there not various bodies of knowledge quite independent of one another, each forming an epistemological core? In short, is it necessary to regard that part of truth which is known as one connected whole of knowledge? For instance, astronomy and ethics might be said to represent the knowledge of two parts of truth, which so far as knowledge goes are separate from each other. The answer to these two questions leads back to a consideration of the structure of truth.

If truth were a mere network of relations, various parts of the network might be known while the relations between these known parts might be unknown, thus making knowledge consist of many distinct groups of relations. This probably represents the status of knowledge, and even the conception of knowledge, as it was in the early development of thought. But, as has been shown, truth has rather the character of a structure and is conditioned by its foundation. The relation of knowledge to truth must then be considered as a relation to truth, as a system of relations centered in a core. And this logical core must in no way be regarded as identical with the epistemological core. To say that truth involves a logical core means that all the relations composing truth are subject to certain necessary conditions, certain fundamental relations. These conditions are either conditions presupposed and implied by all truth or they are conditions presupposed and implied by various special systems of truth. Now since all truth is conditioned by the logical core, not only the relations included under the *abc* of knowledge but also those covered by the *x* are conditioned by it. The *x* is thus a function of the logical core, and as the logical core is, in its most fundamental features, part of positive knowledge, the *x* is in some degree known. At least it may be said that it is known that there is an *x*, and that some of its conditions are known. In other words, the *x*, that part of truth not yet known, being a function of the logical core, and the logical core being included in the epistemological core, the *x* is a function of the *abc* or of the epistemological core. It cannot therefore be maintained that in any stage of knowledge truth can be divided into two parts, one part known and the other part not yet known, as if these two parts were unrelated. Because truth is centered in a core the *abc* and the *x* of knowledge are intimately related, and not only is the relation between them conditioned by the structure of truth, but the whole unity of knowledge is conditioned by this structure.

It may of course be objected that to say that the *x* is known in part is the same as to say that the *x* so far as it is known is part of the *abc* and therefore not part of the *x*, that it is inconsistent to regard the *x* as in any sense known. The contradiction here is merely formal. It may be better to reserve the term *x* for that which is not yet known, not yet actually determined in knowledge. The real issue cuts more deeply. Every truth, every relation in every special system of truth, is conditioned by certain fundamental relations; even these fundamental relations are so conditioned. Whether the relations fall within the *abc* or the *x* of knowledge is immaterial, they are conditioned by the logical core. Therefore, if the logical core is included in the epistemological core some of the conditions of all truth are known. Consequently all truth is known as to its general relational form and as to some of its fundamental conditions. It is all known in its general structure but not in its detail. Knowledge then may have a grasp on the general outline of truth without knowing every specific relation. It may be wise to reserve the term *x* to cover these specific relations which are not yet known, but it ought now to be clear that there is no *x* absolutely unknown in any stage of knowledge. The *x* at any stage is conditioned, is pointed to, is suggested by the known; it is essentially a function of both the logical core and the epistemological core.

As has been already pointed out, truth involves both definiteness and indefiniteness. Knowledge of space as the condition of the known configuration of the contents of any part of space suggests through the conception of space further contents in other parts of space without any suggestion as to the detail of these further contents. Space thus conditions the known and the unknown contents. It is the definite formal condition of all its contents but is indefinite with respect to the particular configuration of the contents. Here, it could be said, space as the known conditions the *x* or the unknown, and the known contents of space suggest further contents which are unknown. The known moral law may suggest a form for all moral acts though only some of those moral acts may be known, the others being indefinite and unknown with respect to the particular factors not defined by the law. Because of direction in the relational form a known *aRb* may point to an unknown *bRc*. The relational form and the fundamental relations of identity, difference, unity, plurality, and systematic order give definite shape and outline to all truth, and as known fundamental forms of relations, as falling within the epistemological core, they yield knowledge of all that is known and is to be known. The logical core then makes it possible for the epistemological core to have a definite view and perspective of all truth while leaving indefinite and thus not including the detail of all its relations. In this way knowledge has access to truth, not through mere addition of truth to truth, or relation to relation, but by starting with a perspective or plan of truth as a whole and then filling in its contents.

The relation of knowledge to truth will become clearer through a consideration of the procedure of knowledge. In any consideration of the progress of knowledge three important matters must now be borne in mind: the relation of knowledge to the logical core, its relation to the epistemological core, and its relation to the object to be determined. The logical core includes the necessary conditions of truth and therefore of all that is to be determined in the progress of knowledge. It suggests the general plan of truth and points to its totality. This unity in the core of truth is of the greatest importance: on it depends the whole systematization of knowledge. Philosophy owes much to Plato and Kant for having made it the cornerstone of thought. The epistemological core includes knowledge of the logical core, of the general outline of truth, and of such detail of this outline as has already been determined. No doubt more still remains to be known of the logical core. Logical research may throw new light upon it, but enough of its character is known to make clear that it is fundamental in the epistemological core. Some detail must also be included in the core of knowledge as a base or starting point for the determination of further knowledge. In fact, inclusion of the logical core without such detail would not be sufficient because a bare outline would be a form without content, and without some content there would be no suggestion as to any particular system of truth. The logical core may suggest definite general conditions but it is indefinite and ambiguous with respect to the more special relations. Some special relations must be known in order to suggest the more special lines for research. Historically, the intuition or conception of special relations arose prior to the conception of necessary conditions, but no thoroughgoing conception of knowledge is possible without conceptions of both. The problem of knowledge is the problem of filling out the detail, the special relations of the epistemological core, or to put it more technically, it is the problem of determining for knowledge the *x* of knowledge, that part of truth which is not yet known. To determine the *x* is to bring it within the fold of the *abc*. As the *x* is inexhaustible, truth being unlimited in range, the determining of the *x* is a dynamic procedure and a procedure without end. To determine the *x* a method is necessary, but this method must be consistent with the unity of truth as expressed in the logical core and with the system of positive knowledge as the starting point, the epistemological core, and with the *x* or object of knowledge as a function of both the logical and epistemological cores.

One method of determining the *x* is to trace out the implications of positive knowledge, that is, to move forward from positive knowledge to further truth implied by positive knowledge, or to reduce such possible further truth to the fundamental conditions and postulates of the logical core. This is called the method of deduction; it is used to some extent in all research, and in the sciences of mathematics and logic it is the primary method. But where truths and relations are not implicative this method is of no avail. The method of hypothesis must then be used. According to this method a truth is projected or set up hypothetically and then tested with respect to its relation to positive knowledge, to its consistency with and relevancy to the epistemological core. The atomic theory and the law of action and reaction are good examples of truths determined by this method, a method which has been especially fruitful in all branches of physical science. If an hypothesis conforms to the conditions of positive knowledge and at the same time enlarges it by unifying and connecting its detail, the hypothesis is regarded as a theory and is then considered as belonging to the body of positive knowledge. As part of the epistemological core it is a basis for further hypotheses, for further determination of the *x*. If, however, in the progress of knowledge new theories or truths appear which enlarge upon or run counter to any accepted theory, that theory may be discarded as inadequate or as no longer holding, though it may still be regarded as true for a particular stage in knowledge. In astronomy the Ptolemaic system was true for the stage of knowledge in the fourteenth century, the Copernican system for the stage of knowledge from the sixteenth century to the twentieth century, and now in the present stage of knowledge a new system seems to be brewing. That detail already determined by knowledge must be redetermined as knowledge advances means, first, that knowledge at any one stage is not knowledge of complete truth, secondly, that as knowledge advances readjustments must be made, and yet, thirdly, that knowledge at any one stage is true for that stage. Thus knowledge advances both by deduction and by hypothesis, but because of the nature of the hypothetical method knowledge always remains incomplete while aiming at completeness.

The place of error in relation to knowledge may now be made clear. Apart from errors which might be called mere mistakes, such as inaccuracy in multiplication or failure to take account of all the factors involved in a problem, it may be said that on the one hand the possibility of error lies in the nature of the structure of truth, and that on the other hand there is no absolute standard in knowledge with respect to which it may be measured. Part of truth does not define the whole of truth, therefore knowledge of a part is indefinite and ambiguous with respect to the rest; but if error is thus made possible it cannot be overcome by comparing the part with the absolute whole of truth. As there is no concrete whole of truth given in knowledge, no hypothetical idea can be measured by it, no positive knowledge can be corrected by it. The only standard with which the truth of any stage of knowledge can be compared is the standard of some succeeding stage. Therefore, as positive knowledge at any stage may not be judged erroneous with respect to itself, it can only be judged erroneous or at least inadequate with respect to a succeeding stage. Though in its progress knowledge aims at completeness or totality, its infinitely far-off goal can never be reached. The determination of error can then lie only in the progress of knowledge. There is therefore not only a place for error in the structure of truth but also a place for its determination in knowledge.

Enough has been said to make clear the general character of knowledge, its procedure, and the relation of error to it, but now the full significance of the relation of knowledge to truth must be considered. Though the relational structure of truth with its logical core suggests an infinite and inexhaustible system of truth, knowledge at any stage is always limited; it seems to be a contact or identification of the mind with a part of truth. Hence it is a point of view, a perspective, truth seen from a particular angle. It may be conceived of either statically as given positive knowledge, or dynamically as expanding knowledge, as moving forward from stage to stage, as gradually determining the *x*. The dynamic conception would seem to be more vital and more complete than the static conception, the latter representing only a phase, an abstraction, one stage, in the more complicated dynamic procedure of determining the *x*. Furthermore, the dynamic conception includes a place for error in knowledge as it also points toward a more complete knowledge, toward the totality of truth suggested by the logical core. Though the dynamic conception expresses more fully the relation of knowledge to truth, the dynamic procedure can never reach its goal, the complete determination of the *x*. So knowledge, even conceived dynamically, must always be limited. Knowledge being limited, and all truth to which reference can be made being known truth, the question may be asked as to whether truth may not after all be knowledge and subject to the conditions and limitations of knowledge. As every truth which can be mentioned is knowledge, as nothing can be referred to, not even the *x*, which is not at least formally knowledge, and as the fullest imaginable expansion of knowledge is of truth seen from a point of view, must not truth be conceived as essentially a perspective? The question may be made more general if it be asked, which is the more fundamental, truth or knowledge? Is truth a function of knowledge or is knowledge a phase of truth? If truth is a function of knowledge, then it is only a series of perspectives or an expanding perspective, while if knowledge is a phase of truth, truth exceeds knowledge and is more than the perspectives of knowledge.

The view that truth is an expanding perspective and therefore esentially knowledge may be called epistemological idealism, and the view that truth extends beyond knowledge and that knowledge can never encompass it may be called epistemological realism. The epistemological realist emphasizes the *x*, the unknown, that part of truth which does not fall within knowledge, and he points out that no matter how far knowledge may progress there will always be an unknown residuum, some truth beyond knowledge. This truth beyond knowledge he regards as not only unknown but also, since it is beyond and outside knowledge, as independent of knowledge. He then comes to think of truth as absolute and unaffected by knowledge, whether conceived of as a whole or in part. The parts may be known or unknown but it is immaterial to them whether they fall within knowledge or not. Knowledge is thus of a part or phase of truth, but it is nothing essential to the relations which compose truth. It proceeds by a kind of addition of truth to truth, by accumulating truth which is unaffected by the accumulating procedure. In contrast with the realist the epistemological idealist emphasizes the relation of the *x* to knowledge. For him the *x* is not so much the unknown as it is that which is to be known. As it is a function of the logical core, and as the logical core is included in the epistemological core, the *x* is at least formally included within knowledge. The *x* is therefore a region outlined in knowledge and to be explored by knowledge. Though it is in detail unknown, it is essentially knowable and significant only for knowledge. Furthermore, the idealist regards the growth of knowledge as not merely a matter of addition, but of addition plus readjustment. And an addition to the *abc* of knowledge may mean change and readjustment within the *abc*. Truth cannot, then, be conceived as divided into two parts, the known and the unknown, with the known encroaching upon the unknown, but must rather be conceived as an expanding known truth, a growing *abc*, the *x* standing for that which the *abc* from its own nature is to become. As it is out of the question to regard truth as something absolute and beyond knowledge, the idealist regards it in some sense as dependent on knowledge. It may not be dependent in the sense that it is made or constructed by the mind, and it may be independent of knowledge in so far as the relations which compose it are dependent on its fundamental structure rather than on its relation to knowledge, but its status is relative to knowledge and it will be found in some respect to be conditioned by knowledge. As dependent on knowledge and with knowledge conceived dynamically it can best be referred to as a growing and changing perspective, as truth "on the march." [24] Thus epistemological realism stands for the independence of truth, with knowledge incidentally accumulating bits of it, while epistemological idealism stands for the dependence of truth on advancing knowledge.

Now as to the relative merits of these two views. To the realist's demand for independence the idealist may maintain that no truth can be referred to which is not relative to knowledge, that the unknown is always a function of the known. The *x*, he will say, is the *x* of knowledge and grounded in known relations; in fact, it could never have been suggested if it were not for certain fundamental relations of the logical core. As the *x*, as well as the *abc*, is a function of the logical core and as the logical core is included in the known then all truth is included in the known, and therefore there is no truth beyond the growing perspective of knowledge. The *x* is merely a factor in the perspective. To ask for more than the perspective is only to ask for more perspective. As a perspective, therefore, truth is not independent but is included in the known.

The idealist is undoubtedly right in so far as he maintains that truth even if infinite and inexhaustible is a function of the logical core and thus relative to known truth, because his view is based on the synthetic and relational conception of truth and on the conception of the logical core as involved in its structure. To characterize truth as a perspective is to

[24] Paul Natorp, *Philosophie, ihr Problem und ihre Probleme* (Göttingen. 1911), p. 34.

regard it as an outline based on the logical core, with some detail determined and some not yet determined. There is no place for anything beyond or independent of this perspective. Furthermore, unless the logical core is to be given up and with it the whole conception of the structure of truth as set forth earlier in this chapter, the growth of knowledge cannot be regarded as an accumulation of independent bits of truth but rather as an expansion of knowledge involving constant readjustment.

But the realist may now suggest a distinction. He may say that the conception of knowledge is ambiguous, that it may mean known truth or the actual knowing of the truth. He may now be willing to admit that all truth is a function of known truth but not that it is a function of the knowing of truth nor that it is in any way conditioned by knowing. Should some idealist hold that truth is made or constructed by the mind, the realist could answer that the trueness of such truth does not depend on its being made or constructed or suggested or thought of by the mind but solely on its having a place in the structure of truth, and it would make no difference whether such truth were a relation included in the logical core or a relation connected with some more special hypothesis or theory. In conceding that all truth may be a function of the known truth, the realist accepts the view that truth must be conceived as an incompleted structure, or as a perspective, but he does insist that it is still essentially a structure and uninfluenced by its relation to the mind. Accordingly truth must be regarded as known structure but not as structure due in any way to its being known. In other words, epistemological idealism is correct with regard to the incompleteness and growing character of truth while epistemological realism is correct with regard to its structural character.

Realism might then seem to be in the stronger position, and indeed if knowledge contributes nothing to truth except to bring out its incompleteness idealism might be set aside, because the incompleteness of truth might possibly be shown to be a phase of its structure. But it is just this incompleteness of truth which idealism regards as due to knowledge.

For idealism the incompleteness of truth, its perspective character, that is, its limitation, is conditioned by the limitations of knowledge. After consideration of various factors involved in the relation of knowledge to truth the final issue as to which is the more fundamental comes down to the question as to whether the structure of truth is in any way dependent on knowledge. Both epistemological realism and epistemological idealism accept the view of logical idealism that all truth is a function of the logical core, and they agree that truth is not a construction of the mind, but they disagree as to whether or not knowledge contains any condition which affects truth.

The realist insists upon the independence of the structure of truth for two reasons. In the first place he would hold that any particular relation or group of relations such as the equality of 2 plus 2 and 4, or the structure of a molecule of oxygen, or the shape of a house, is not determined by the mind which happens to know it and therefore has a status independent of knowledge. And secondly he would hold that any such relation is a function of the logical core and belongs to a system of relations not involving or being determined by mind or knowledge. The structure of truth would then seem to stand on its own feet and to be unaffected by knowledge. But how about the distinction between the *abc* and the *x*, between the truth determined and the truth not yet determined? This distinction cannot be made on the basis of structure alone without reference to knowledge, and yet all structure, any group of relations to which the mind has access, involves, suggests, or points to further structure or relations not yet determined in knowledge. If truth cannot be conceived of as something given absolutely, but only as a growing perspective, as truth "on the march," then as truth "on the march" it implies the "march" of knowledge. The realist is undoubtedly right in maintaining that the structure of truth is not dependent on knowledge, that structure as such is not defined or determined by mind; but if the only structure which the mind may intuit or of which the mind may become aware is a changing or growing structure, then, unless consideration is given to that which governs the movement and the growth of the structure, namely knowledge, the whole story is not told.

This close relation of truth to knowledge has led some thinkers to regard truth as essentially the structure of knowledge and therefore as knowledge, as for instance Cohen and Natorp, who bring all truth, including the logical core, under knowledge (*Erkenntnis*) or thought (*Denken*).[25] It is not their intention to make truth either as structure or as conditioned by fundamental logical principles in any way dependent on mind, but they do feel that truth can hardly be referred to except as an object or principle or factor of knowledge. In this work truth has been treated — in so far as it is a structure or system of relations — as primary, and therefore as prior to knowledge, and in so far as it is conditioned by the logical core, as not dependent on knowledge. But it has also been shown that while knowledge may be regarded as secondary no full conception of truth can be given without consideration of its relation to knowledge, and for two reasons. First, no truth can be considered or referred to which is not in some way known or does not come within the purview of knowledge or is not accessible to mind. In other words, no reference can be made to any truth without mind to make such reference; truth cannot be known to be true unless there is knowledge of it. Knowledge cannot be escaped when truth is concerned, even if the nature of truth's structure may not be defined by knowledge. And secondly, no truth can be pursued, no search for it can be made, except on the basis of truth already known, that is, the truth to be determined must be suggested by the detail known, by the *abc*. Not only then does truth involve knowledge because it involves presence to mind but also because the lines of truth to be determined are relative to that which is determined.

To make clearer the relation of truth to knowledge, three factors must be distinguished, truth, knowledge, and mind. Now it is not possible on the one hand to identify knowledge

[25] Cohen, *Logik der reinen Erkenntniss*, pp. 1–64; Natorp, *Die logischen Grundlagen der exakten Wissenschaften*, pp. 1–97.

with mind in the sense that it is merely an intuition or an awareness of truth on the part of mind, nor is it possible to identify it with truth as just the content of which the mind is aware. Neither access to truth by mind nor structure of truth which the mind may intuit is sufficient to account for knowledge. To emphasize mind and to speak of knowledge as mind's intuition or awareness may cover what is meant by knowing but hardly what is generally understood by knowledge. But if knowledge is referred to the structure of truth, then it ought to be possible to speak of truth and knowledge as if they were identical. This however cannot be done. For instance, while it would be possible to speak of the configuration of the material forming the interior of the earth as partly known and as partly unknown or to be known, it would not be possible to speak of it as partly true and as partly untrue or not yet true or to be true. The dynamic character of knowledge, as the encroachment of the *abc* upon the *x*, makes it impossible to identify knowledge with truth when truth is conceived of as structure. The structure being the primary dimension of truth, knowledge may be regarded as a kind of second dimension distinct from structure. As long as it is not possible to attain to any absolute truth, whether considered as a whole or in part, truth cannot be conceived except under the dynamic conditions of knowledge. Knowledge as well as structure is essential to a theory of truth; neither the primary dimension nor the secondary dimension can be dispensed with.

Knowledge then stands for the dynamic aspect of truth. As the epistemological core, including the general outline of the logical core and the detail already known, suggests the further detail which is to be filled in, knowledge may be said to suggest the problems to which truth as structure is the answer. In other words, knowledge covers the problematic side of truth. It is common to speak of the problem or the problems of knowledge while truth is regarded as the solution of the questions raised in the problems. As the *x* of knowledge is both a function of the *abc* and a symbol of that which is to be known, it may well stand for the problem of knowledge. The *x* is that which is to be known as growing out of that which is known. The dynamic aspect of truth is thus expressed primarily in the problematic side of knowledge. The structure of truth and the *x* of knowledge are the high points in a consideration of a theory of truth. They represent its static and dynamic aspects.

The result with regard to the relation of knowledge to truth may be stated briefly as follows: First of all, logical idealism is accepted so far as the relational character of truth is concerned, as also with regard to its centering in and being a function of the logical core. Truth's structure is essentially connected and unified. Then secondly, epistemological realism is accepted so far as the structure of truth is recognized as not dependent on knowledge, as not merely an expanding perspective. As more than an expanding perspective it must not be conceived of as something absolute and unrelated to knowledge, but rather as a structure not determined by knowledge. Finally, epistemological idealism is accepted in so far as truth is recognized to be the object and objective of knowledge and essentially related to it. Epistemological idealism so understood does not imply that the structure of truth is constructed or made true by knowledge, it simply means that apart from the intuition of truth or the contact of mind with the structure of truth, apart from the growing perspective and the "march" of knowledge, apart from the problematic character of knowledge, the *abc–x* relation, truth would be a vain and incomplete conception. Epistemological realism is here little more than a concession to logical idealism, a recognition of the primacy of the structure of truth and its unity. It might therefore be sufficient to characterize the position above outlined as that of combined logical and epistemological idealism, the structural character of truth being primary and the problematic character of knowledge being secondary, but both being fundamental and essential.

On the basis of the foregoing outline of the relation of knowledge to truth, the more special problems of knowledge in their relation to the more special systems of truth may now be considered. The problems of knowledge are many and varied, in fact, as many as there are questions which may be asked. They do, however, group themselves into certain fundamental problems. They may even be classed under one fundamental problem, the problem of knowledge, but it has not been easy to group them under one general problem without loss or neglect of that which gives them their specific character. Evidence for the diversity of problems is to be found in the variety of sciences and branches of philosophy. Instead of the *x* of knowledge there is the logical *x*, the mathematical *x*, the physical *x*, the moral *x*, the psychological *x*, etc., and philosophy has not yet succeeded in bringing these problems under one fundamental problem except in so far as they are conditioned by the central logical core, the formal logical principles. Since this work is concerned with the psychological problem it is important to take account of the relation of that problem not only to the general problem of knowledge but also to the other more special problems. It will then be necessary to ask what the fundamental problems are and how they are grouped in the present status of knowledge.

There are four general types of problems: (1) logical problems, (2) imaginary problems, (3) real problems, and (4) teleological problems.

(1) Logical problems, or the problems of the logical core, are the problems connected with the fundamental relations of all truth. They are concerned with the relations of quality, quantity, order, etc., with the development of such conceptions as that of class, contradiction, continuity, infinity, and other related conceptions. In the recent overhauling of logic and mathematics much has been done by way of clarification and solution of the problems associated with these conceptions. Not only should the problems of the central core, of the *sine qua non* of all knowledge, but also those connected with the foundation of the more special systems of truth be regarded as logical problems, such for instance as problems as to the *sine qua non* of the physical world or of the moral world. As these problems also involve consideration of the details of the more special systems of knowledge they tend to

fall under the types of problems other than the logical ones, but as they involve also universal relations they have a place among logical problems. In other words, although logical problems are not unconnected with the other types of problems they include a universal content which may be developed as pure knowledge irrespective of and in part independently of the other types.

(2) Imaginary problems are problems involving further details than logical problems but details suggested by the imagination. The problems are chosen rather arbitrarily, consonant to be sure with the logical core but not related in any fundamental way to the real or teleological worlds. Examples of such problems are to be found in logical and mathematical systems based upon freely chosen postulates, in purely ideal moral systems or states, or in conceptions of possible realities beyond and unrelated to the known world. Inconsistent systems might possibly be here included, but research in these systems would tend to eliminate the inconsistencies. The value of these problems and the imaginary systems with which they are connected is largely to be found in the light which they throw upon real and teleological systems by way of contrast, and in the suggestion that comes from them as to the wide range of possibilities and possible problems conditioned by the logical core.

(3) Real problems are those connected with reality, existence, actuality, fact, with that which is as distinct from that which ought to be or from that which is merely possible. They are conditioned by the logical core, but they involve detail not included in it. The detail cannot be regarded as something arbitrarily chosen but as something to be accepted and taken into account in knowledge. In a sense, it is given in knowledge and intuited by the mind, but not as something other than truth with which it is to be contrasted. It should be conceived of as among the relations composing truth and as a function of the logical core. So far as it is known, it may be said to belong to the *abc* of knowledge, and so far as it is to be known, to belong to the *x* of knowledge. It may be convenient to speak of this detail as phenomena or appearances

to distinguish it from the relations of the logical core and imaginary systems. As phenomena are a function of knowledge the problem arises as to their determination. The problem of reality or existence is the problem as to the appearances, as to a system of truth inclusive of all appearances and their conditions.

In the present status of knowledge, the most successful attempt at solution of the problem of reality or appearances is to be found in the truth of physical science. The physical world may well be defined as the world of space–time including space–time and all that is spatial and temporal. Geometry, mechanics, astronomy, physics, chemistry, biology, all contribute toward a solution of the physical problem. With many thinkers the term science has come to mean knowledge of the physical world. In modern times physical research has opened up new vistas and new problems, and many have felt that all real problems will be solved by its methods. Yet in spite of this success, beside the physical problem two other problems of reality must be considered, the ontological problem and the psychological problem.

The ontological problem like the physical problem is concerned with a synthesis of truth which includes all phenomena and their conditions. It takes account of the spatio-temporal character of appearances but raises the question as to whether the conditions of appearances may not imply something supertemporal and superspatial. It raises the question as to whether there is an ultimate and eternal framework of reality, and as to whether the outline of this framework can in any way be determined. Is reality a definite concrete order conditioned by the logical core and conditioning the appearances, something ultimate and all-inclusive? A solution of this problem is most certainly difficult if not impossible. From the earliest days philosophers have tried to solve this problem, but with little or no success. Of the many ontologies which are discussed today none is accepted as a part of positive knowledge. At best they are regarded as possible hypotheses. Their value is largely negative. The ontological problem is suggestive both of the limitation of knowledge and of its infinite possibilities. Though it adds little to knowledge, it does yield perspective and is therefore a genuine problem.

The psychological problem is the problem as to mind and its nature. Mind is existent, it is a phenomenon of some sort and therefore belongs to the real world of appearances. Just what the mind is is still very much an open question. Some thinkers regard it as a phase of the physical world, as having its place somewhere in the spatio-temporal order, and they regard psychology as a branch of physical science, of biology. Others regard it as something non-spatial if not non-temporal, and therefore as not identifiable with the physical world. Such questions as the following may serve to make clear this issue: Is the sensation of a color or a tone a phase of the physical world or something distinct from that world? Are all perceptions which include a spatial characteristic identifiable with the space of the physical system? Is a mind which on the basis of memory looks back over the past something supertemporal? Or is a mind which can think logical or mathematical formulae non-temporal? Again, if it be granted that appearances appear or are in some way intuited, is it possible to regard the appearing or the intuiting as a physical function in space–time? Those who believe that there are phases of phenomena which cannot be included in the physical world hold that mind is something distinct from the spatio-temporal medium and that psychology is distinct from physical science. If mind is not physical, or even if only the question is asked as to its being other than physical, the psychological problem is raised. In modern thought this problem has been most decidedly raised, and this work is an attempt to clarify and to offer some solution to the problem. While as compared with the ontological problem it is less vague and has something definite to offer, it has nothing of the clarity and determinateness of the physical problem.

Though the real problems may be much further ramified, they center in the three concepts of space–time, ultimate reality, and mind. Through them three fundamental problems relative to phenomena are defined.

(4) Teleological problems are problems connected with

purpose, end, ideal, with that which ought to be as distinct from that which is. They are problems with respect to the definition of ends to be attained. An end or purpose may vary all the way from being the goal of the most trivial desire to the synthesis of the highest possible moral or aesthetic ideal. There are however three kinds of teleological problems which ought to be mentioned.

First of all there are the problems of technique, the problems connected with the adjustment of means to ends, the practical problems of finding the proper conditions to fulfill purposes. Such sciences as medicine and electrical engineering are concerned with problems of this type. But these problems of technique are very varied and cannot be organized under any one system of truth except so far as they fall within the general system of knowledge or are unified in a moral system. They naturally lead to a consideration of the moral problem.

Secondly, then, there is the moral problem. This is the problem as to the unity and organization of ends and purposes themselves, the central teleological problem. It is the problem of the ideal end of all ends, the problem as to what the system of all ends should be. As ends are the expression of wills or are phases of will, the moral problem is also the problem of the organization of all wills so far as they have their being in ends. A body of truth giving foundation or unity to all ends and wills is called an ethical system and is the basis of the solution of the moral problem. The moral problem is one of the most important and far-reaching of the philosophical problems. All human activities, all technique, and even knowledge itself as a human activity fall within its scope. It is the problem *par excellence* of the unity of human ideals.

Thirdly, there is the aesthetic problem. It is the problem as to the nature and criteria of the beautiful, as to beauty as an end or ideal, as perfection of composition or organization in nature and in art. This problem has been very freely and fully discussed in modern thought but is still the least well defined of all the fundamental philosophical problems; yet it is a problem which holds a distinct place among teleological problems.

The four general types of problems have suggested eight fundamental groups of problems: Logical problems, imaginary or unreal problems, the physical problem, the ontological problem, the psychological problem, problems of technique, the moral problem, and the aesthetic problem. This grouping of fundamental problems rounds out the conception of truth. It not only suggests the basic problems and so defines the various systems of truth, but it also helps to make clear the problematic and dynamic side of the knowledge of truth. It represents the present status of the *abc* and the *x* of knowledge. The problems suggested may give rise with the progress of knowledge to further fundamental problems and sub-problems, and again some of the problems may be brought together under more general problems and thus unified under larger systems of truth. For instance, just as the physical problem and the psychological problem were clearly distinguished in early modern times, so further problematic distinctions may be made, and it is also quite within the range of possibility that as the result of future research these two problems may be united under one basic problem. But however the grouping of problems may develop, it is important in the understanding of the psychological problem, the problem of this work, to understand the present status of the grouping. In an attempt to offer some solution of the psychological problem and to determine its place in the system of truth and knowledge, its relation to the other problems cannot be neglected. Therefore, special consideration will be given to its relation to some of the other problems, particularly to the logical problem, the physical problem, the moral problem, and the ontological problem. To define mind in the system of truth, to determine its place in knowledge, involves the problematic situation and the interrelation of the various problems of knowledge.

As a condition to the determination of the psychological problem a theory of the structure and knowledge of truth has been set forth. Before this problem is considered, some possible objections to the theory should be met and a summary of the chief theses involved in the theory should be given.

As to the objections: first of all, objection may be made to the conception of truth as the fundamental conception. So far as mere terminology is concerned this objection is of little importance. It would be quite possible to substitute for the term truth some other term, such as system, system of relations, body of propositions, world, knowledge, reality, being, or any other term, provided such term were to mean what is meant by truth in this work, namely a system of relations centered in a core and related to knowledge. But with respect to the meaning and content of truth it might be said that such concepts as being, entity, reality, existence, and again such concepts as proposition, judgment, experience, and even consciousness, are more fundamental than the concept of truth. There are, however, three reasons for holding truth to be more fundamental than the other conceptions. The philosophy expressed in this work holds in the first place that synthesis, relation, connection, or system is basic, and that analysis or separation is not primary however valuable it may be as an aid to synthesis. Now such concepts as being and entity, which are suggestive of analysis, are not so appropriate as is the concept of truth to a synthetic philosophy. Secondly, this philosophy recognizes a variety of problems conditioned in their solution by a central body of principles. The concepts of reality and existence do not express the full systematic conception of the relation of the core to the problems. They stand rather for one group of problems. There being problems not only of that which is real and which exists, but also of that which is not real but ought to be or ought to exist, and of that which is imaginary and not real at all, the conception of reality or existence cannot well apply to the whole system of problems but rather to one group of problems, whereas the concept of truth, being systematic, can well cover all. Thirdly, this philosophy recognizes an objective structure, and while the structure is not absolute nor unrelated to knowledge it is not conceived as based upon any mental concept. Therefore, all concepts which suggest or point to mind must be excluded as fundamental concepts. The concept of proposition may seem objective, but it is hardly so objective as truth, nor is it so systematic. It may be conceived of either as a verbal expression of truth, or as expressing a unit of truth, or as a relation belonging to a system of relations. In the former case it is no fundamental concept, and in the latter case, though it points to a system, it is not so expressive of a system as is the conception of truth. A judgment has objective reference but it also has reference to the judging mind and is therefore not so suitable as the conception of truth. As a concept of a system of relations experience is even more ambiguous, always connoting the experiencer as well as the experienced, and consciousness, though often thought to be the source of synthesis, is essentially subjective or mental in reference. The concept of truth has the advantage of suggesting structure and system while at the same time avoiding implication of absolute systems and subordination to mental principles as compared with other concepts.

Then it may be objected that relations have been given a more fundamental place than universals, and it may be claimed that a consideration of classes, fundamental concepts, and categories should come before a consideration of relations. But it should be noted that relations have not been given higher rank than universals; they have been given equal rank. All relations are universals as all universals are relations. A universal as a concept, that is, in intension, is essentially a relation; and as defining the members of a class, in extension, it is also a relation, a unity of the class. The classing, grouping, and organizing of relations in a system and the recognition of the fundamental relations composing the logical core have not been neglected, and nowhere in the development of the relational theory of truth has relation been given precedence over the universal, even if it is unusual to give an account of relation before giving an account of the universal conceptions and categories. If relation has not been given precedence, the universal on the other hand has not been given higher rank than relation and regarded as more extensive. Analytic logic has generally assumed the terminal theory or the terminal-relational theory of truth. Terms have been considered at least as of equal rank with relations and therefore the logic of classes, of universals, has come before the logic of relations. But now, with the acceptance of the relational theory of truth and the treating of terms as terminals of relation and therefore essentially as relational, the logic of classes becomes the logic of classes of relations. Relation, then, as the primary and fundamental character of truth, may well be considered at the outset of any study of truth, and it may be given, if not higher rank, at least equal rank with the universal, because it is the essential content of the universal.

One further objection should be considered. It may be said that truth is essentially structure and does not need knowledge as a kind of second dimension, that to introduce the conception of knowledge is to lead the way to subjectivism. The relation of truth to knowledge and mind will be considered in a later chapter, but it may be pointed out here that the structure of truth is in no way endangered by its relation to knowledge, since structure is primary and in no way dependent on mind. Yet the reference to knowledge in a conception of truth is unavoidable. As absolute truth is unattainable whether considered as the absolute totality of all truth or as the final character of any part of truth, nothing is left but the truth relative to the stages of knowledge, the expanding truth in the *abc–x* relation. Such truth is the fullest attainable truth, but it implies expansion, and because it is synthetic and not merely additive it implies constant reorganization. How such truth could be defined irrespective of its relation to knowledge it is hard to see, although its structure is not determined by knowledge. The second dimension of truth, knowledge, is merely its dynamic dimension. It stands for the constant renovating but not the renovations of the structure. It expresses the limitation and expansion beyond the limitation of available truth. Thus as relative to knowledge truth is not a final concretion but rather a mixture of actual and possible structure.

The summary of the chief theses of this chapter may be given as follows:

(1) Truth is fundamentally synthetic or relational, not analytic or disconnected. This conception is derived from the coherence theory so far as it suggests systematic coherence and connection but not so far as it implies either the absolute whole as the sole truth or the internality of relations. In opposition to the terminal and terminal-relational theories this relational theory of truth means that truth is essentially a system or nexus of relations of relations, with possible ultimate terms or terminals internal to the relations, and it makes relation consist of a unity involving specific character, terminals, and sense or direction. And as relational, truth is formally the most fundamental and comprehensive of conceptions.

(2) Truth is centered in a core or body of fundamental or necessary relations of which all further relations are a function. The synthetic character of relation, the more specific types of relation, and implication in relational systems all point to this core, which forms the foundation of the structure or ordered system of all truth, and which consists of such general logical relations as identity, difference, class, unity, plurality, number, order, etc., and of those relations which are the presuppositions and conditions of the more special branches of truth. Although all truth implies the logical core and an outline defined by that core, it is unlimited and not determined in all its details by the universal relations of the core. The relational content of truth thus reveals system and order based on, though not fully determined by, fundamental relations.

(3) Truth is related to knowledge, as is suggested by the intuitional theory. Knowledge as a kind of access to or intuition of truth, on the one hand, is limited and hence not of ultimate truth; and on the other hand, as a function of the mind, it does not construct or produce truth. As knowledge is dynamic and expansive, it implies a moving perspective of truth, advancing from stage to stage, each stage being expressed by the *abc–x* relation. The *abc* stands for positive knowledge both of the core and of further detail, that which

is already determined, and the *x* for the inexhaustible field which is to be determined. Knowledge of truth moves forward by implication and by hypothesis, and as the truth at each stage may involve reorganization and reconstruction, as the procedure is not merely additive, no stage of truth can be regarded in any sense as final. Yet truth "on the march" is the only available truth, and as such it is essentially related to knowledge as a kind of second dimension. The conception of truth then implies both consideration of its relational structure and reference to the procedure of knowledge.

(4) Error, the importance of which is brought out by the correspondence theory, is due – according to the coherence or relational theory – not to any falling short of a fixed standard or ultimate whole of truth, but rather to the indefiniteness in its composition and structure as relative to the various stages in knowledge. The synthesis of truth at any stage of knowledge cannot fully determine the truth of any further stage, and therefore may be in error in trying to project the content of that further stage; but the further stage may correct the error of the earlier stage and so determine error by serving as a kind of relative standard. Each stage is thus a synthesis of truth unto itself but may be an erroneous synthesis with respect to some further stage of synthesis. Error is possible through the dimension of knowledge.

(5) The problematic character of knowledge is a result of the expansion of truth in knowledge. The *x* as a function of the logical core and of the detail of positive knowledge represents that which is to be determined; but as positive knowledge branches out into more special systems, so the *x* of knowledge as a function of these systems divides into corresponding problems. There are four general types of problems – logical, imaginary, real, and teleological. The real problems divide into three sub-problems – the physical problem, the ontological problem, the psychological problem; and the teleological problems divide also into three sub-problems – the technical problem, the moral problem, the aesthetic problem.

Now back to the problem of psychology.

CHAPTER III

MIND

THE SCIENCE OF PSYCHOLOGY is generally distinguished from the so-called normative sciences of logic, ethics, and aesthetics. It is distinguished from them as being a science of the real as opposed to the ideal. It is said to be concerned with actual facts or realities, whereas the normative sciences measure the facts and realities according to some standard.[1] Pfänder says: "Logic considers thinking in respect to truth; it brings a measure to bear on thought and separates off the correct from the incorrect thinking; while psychology investigates thinking with respect to its real nature and law, it applies no measure to it"; he does not ask "whether that which is held to be true or false is really true or false." [2] McDougall defines psychology as "the positive science of the conduct of living creatures," "the science which attempts to describe and explain the conduct of men and other living creatures, and is not concerned with questions as to what their conduct ought to be." [3] What conduct ought to be is left to ethics. Psychology is concerned with the fact and ethics with the ideal of conduct. In the same way psychology is opposed to aesthetics, the former having to do with the contemplation of the beautiful and the latter with its nature.[4] Psychology may therefore include within its sphere actual thought, conduct, and contemplation, but not the ideals of the true, the good, and the beautiful, except in so far as they are actually embodied in reality. To be sure, it is possible to find thinkers who slur over this distinction — as, for instance, Fowler, who

[1] George Frederick Stout, *A Manual of Psychology* (New York, 1899), pp. 4–6.

[2] Alexander Pfänder, *Einführung in die Psychologie* (Leipzig, 1904), p. 48; see also Wilhelm Wundt, *Logik* (3rd ed., Stuttgart, 1906–08), I, 1–2; Francis Herbert Bradley, *The Principles of Logic* (London, 1883), pp. 2–3; Leonard Trelawney Hobhouse, *The Theory of Knowledge* (London, 1896), pp. 4–5.

[3] William McDougall, *Physiological Psychology* (London, 1905), p. 1.

[4] James Sully, *The Human Mind* (New York, 1892), II, 360.

says: "Thoughts or the results of Thinking" become "the subject of a science with a distinct name, Logic, which is thus a subordinate branch of the wider science, Psychology." [5] Yet it is usual to find psychology contrasted with the sciences of the ideal and made distinctly a science of the factual.

On the one hand, this distinction between psychology and the normative sciences is of importance in placing psychology among the sciences of the real, and therefore in differentiating its problem from the problems of teleological and imaginary systems as well as from those concerned with logical structure; on the other hand, it leads to the recognition of the superior place of logic as the science of criteria and fundamentals and of ethics and aesthetics as sciences of standards and values. It is, however, unfortunate to group logic with ethics and aesthetics, since logic is not primarily a science of norms or standards but rather a science of structure, of the structural foundations of all sciences, including ethics and aesthetics, whereas ethics and aesthetics as teleological sciences, as sciences of value, are more special sciences dealing with the norms and standards of conduct and beauty. Furthermore, it is misleading to refer to logic as a science of thinking or thought, because these terms suggest mind and are more properly psychological, logic being the science of truth rather than of thought. This ambiguous use of the term thought may easily lead to treating logic as dependent on psychology. But to subordinate logic to psychology is to make an upper story of a building support its foundation. Logic as a science of the criteria or the fundamental principles of the structure of all truth can hardly be a phase of psychology, which is concerned with one branch of the structure. In spite of these difficulties, and in spite of the lack of clearness in the differentiation of psychology from the normative sciences as generally stated, this differentiation has outstanding value in limiting psychology to a place among the sciences of the real or

[5] Thomas Fowler, *The Elements of Deductive Logic* (10th ed., Oxford, 1892), pp. 2–3; see also Guido Villa, *Contemporary Psychology*, translated by Harold Manacorda (London, 1903), pp. 81–83; George Trumbull Ladd, *Psychology Descriptive and Explanatory* (3rd ed., New York, 1896), p. 11.

factual, thereby defining its character in one very essential way.

Among the sciences of the real, three fundamental problems and therefore three fundamental kinds of sciences have been distinguished — physical, ontological, and psychological. It is hardly necessary here to consider the distinction between psychology and ontology. Ontology has to do with the ultimate framework of reality, while psychology is concerned with the more special problem of mind. Ontological idealism may seek to identify a mental principle with ultimate reality, but this is no concern of psychology, though it may be of interest in a consideration of the relation of mind to ultimate reality. Ontological definitions of mind such as the "spiritual substance" used by Locke and Berkeley need hardly be considered today as serious conceptions of mind. It is far more important to consider the relation of psychology to physical science.

Since Descartes psychology has often been distinguished from physical science as having to do with a different kind or part of reality or with a different phase of the world. It is thought to be concerned with the internal as contrasted with the external world. The external or physical world being characterized as spatial, the internal world of psychology is said to be non-spatial, though temporal.[6] Höffding says that psychology is the "science of that which thinks, feels, and wills, in contrast with physics as the science of that which moves in space and occupies space," [7] and according to Höfler, physical phenomena appear as spatial, while "all psychical phenomena are non-spatial." [8] "Mental states are thus solely temporal events," [9] as Marvin puts it; they are in time only, while physical events are in both space and time. Psychology is then defined as the science of non-spatial but temporal reality.

[6] Alexander Bain, *The Senses and the Intellect* (4th ed., New York, 1902), p. 1; Sully, *The Human Mind*, I, 7.

[7] Harald Höffding, *Outlines of Psychology*, translated by Mary E. Lowndes (London, 1891), p. 1.

[8] Alois Höfler, *Psychologie* (Vienna, 1897), p. 4.

[9] Walter T. Marvin, *An Introduction to Systematic Philosophy* (New York, 1903), p. 131.

It is easy to see why this definition of psychology has held its ground so long. Its proponents have felt on the one hand that mind is not a physical object and consequently not something to be met with in space, and on the other hand that its activities and functions must go on under the form of time and therefore that mind cannot escape being temporal. The attempt to rescue mind from space may be good as a way of avoiding a materialistic interpretation of mind, but still to leave it in time is to show great lack of discrimination in understanding its nature. To begin with time as a determining conception is impossible without space, because nothing can be determined as in time, or regarded as taking place in time, or referred to any part of time unless it is determined in space, or regarded as taking place in space, or referred to some part of space.[10] Time is therefore useless as the fundamental and definitive conception of psychology. Then, too, there are very few temporal phenomena which are not spatial. If such phenomena are mental they hardly suggest a temporal but non-spatial character of mind. It may be objected, of course, that a feeling of pleasure or a melody is temporal without being spatial, yet to determine the length of time during which a pleasure lasts would involve reference to organic conditions and therefore to an organism, an object in space, and to determine the time, that is, the hour, day, and year in which the melody was performed, would imply also a determination of the place, the concert hall, in which it was performed. In fact, the determination of change involves multiplicity of content, that is, coexistence, and coexistence involves at least some rudimentary conception of space. It is hard to avoid the mechanical pattern of temporal change as the alteration in time of spatial configurations. To try, then, to separate mind from the physical world in space and then to put it in time is virtually to put it back into the physical world again, the world of space–time. The definition of psychology

[10] Paul Natorp, *Einleitung in die Psychologie nach kritischer Methode* (Freiburg, 1888), pp. 62, 67–72; *Allgemeine Psychologie nach kritischer Methode* (Tübingen, 1912), pp. 148–149, 159–168, 254; Hugo Münsterberg, *Grundzüge der Psychologie* (Leipzig, 1900), p. 322.

as a science of non-spatial but temporal reality is therefore inadequate and in unstable equilibrium. Psychology must either become a branch of physical science and determine mind in some way within the space–time system, or, in order to determine the inner nature of mind as distinct from the external or physical world, it must turn to a non-temporal as well as non-spatial conception.

Such a conception is to be found in that of consciousness. But before this conception is considered another definition of psychology should be mentioned, and that is the conception of psychology as the science of the individual as opposed to the over-individual. Here psychology is not characterized so much by its differentiation from the physical sciences as by its intimate relation to them. It has to do not so much with special objects of its own as with a point of view from which the physical world and all truth may be experienced or known. It is defined as the science of the individual, or as the science of any object, reality, or experience so far as it is related to the individual. Avenarius says, the "object of empirical psychology is any experience, . . . as dependent on the individual, in relation to which it . . . is an experience." [11] According to Ward, no particular kind of experience or class of object falls to psychology: "psychology cannot be defined by reference to a special subject-matter as such concrete sciences, for example, as mineralogy and botany can be . . ."; "it must be characterized by the standpoint from which . . . experience is viewed." And its standpoint is, he says, "individualistic." [12]

But to make psychology consist in the study of objects as related to the individual is not to make an adequate definition of psychology unless the individual is further defined. Avenarius' tendency is to regard the individual as determined

[11] Richard Avenarius "Bemerkungen zum Begriff des Gegenstandes der Psychologie," *Vierteljahrschrift für wissenschaftliche Philosophie* (Leipzig), XVIII (1894), 417, see also p. 415; also Oswald Külpe, *Grundriss der Psychologie* (Leipzig, 1893), p. 2.

[12] James Ward, "Psychology," in *Encyclopaedia Britannica* (11th ed., Cambridge, 1911), XXII, 548, and "Psychological Principles," in *Mind* (London and Edinburgh), O.S., VIII (1883), 161–162.

by the brain,[13] and Ebbinghaus and Titchener define it through the whole body or organism.[14] In other words, the individual is defined through part of the world which can be its object or experience. To this Ward is opposed. He says that "the series of feelings" or phenomena which make up experience are not sufficient unless the "subject of these feelings or phenomena" is added. Therefore he makes the individual consist in the "subject of these feelings of phenomena plus the series of feelings or phenomena themselves." [15] The subject or self or ego, which feels, knows, and acts, is for him essential, and he regards the subject–object relation as fundamental to psychology. As Bosanquet explains, "the psychologist deals solely with facts of presentation to particular minds, while the student of natural science neglects this characteristic, and thinks of his objects quite apart from their relation to particular minds." [16] "The ultimate data" of psychology "are therefore," as Stout says, "objects as presented to the individual mind." [17] The individual implies here something more than a part of the world which can be its object or experience, it implies over and above the object or experience a subject or self which is aware of the object or to which the object is presented. Attempts to characterize the individual thus lead in two directions, according to whether the individual is defined through the body or through the mind. If the individual is defined through the body, psychology becomes a branch of physical science; but if through the mind, then psychology holds a place of its own as distinct from physical science.

The tendency to treat psychology as a branch of physical science leads on to functional psychology and behaviorism,

[13] Avenarius, pp. 418–419.

[14] Hermann Ebbinghaus, *Grundzüge der Psychologie* (Leipzig, 1902), I, 7; Edward Bradford Titchener, *A Text-Book of Psychology* (New York, 1911), p. 16; Külpe, *Grundriss der Psychologie*, p. 4.

[15] Ward, "Psychology," in *Encyclopaedia Britannica*, XXII, 550–551, or his "Psychological Principles," *Mind*, O.S., VIII, 466, 470.

[16] Bernard Bosanquet, *Psychology of the Moral Self* (London, 1904), p. 3; see also James Ward, "On the Definition of Psychology," *British Journal of Psychology* (Cambridge), I (1904), 17; Münsterberg, *Grundzüge der Psychologie*, pp. 202–203, 209.

[17] Stout, *A Manual of Psychology*, p. 16.

and will be considered later. The tendency to give psychology a distinct place leads on to those conceptions of mind which make consciousness its central feature. The definition of psychology as "the science which describes and explains the phenomena of consciousness, as such" [18] is characteristic of this tendency. Though there is not unanimity of opinion as to what consciousness is, probably there is no term more suggestive of psychology than the term consciousness. An analysis of this conception or of the various ways in which it is conceived must now be undertaken.

The term consciousness most naturally suggests the relation of knowing or awareness. As a relation it involves terms and may be expressed as something knowing something or something being aware of something. It might be defined as appearing or as experiencing, as an appearance appearing to a knower or an experiencer experiencing an experience. It could also be expressed in the form of a feeler feeling a feeling or of a perceiver perceiving a perception or of a thinker thinking a thought. In general the relation may be spoken of as the subject–object or the ego–content relation. These various forms of expressing this relation throw very little light on its nature. What is meant by the object or content, that of which there is consciousness, a thought or an experience, may be obvious, but the relation of the object to the subject, to that which is aware of it, is not brought out; nor is the nature of the subject or ego itself made clear. This difficulty has made many feel what Angell expresses in saying, "consciousness we can only define in terms of itself. Sensations, ideas, pains, pleasures, acts of memory, imagination, and will – these may serve to illustrate the experiences we mean to indicate by the term; and our best endeavor to construct a successful definition results in some such list, of which we can only say: 'These taken together are what I mean by consciousness.' " [19] Instead of defining consciousness by

[18] Ladd, *Psychology Descriptive and Explanatory*, p. 1; see also Theodor Ziehen, *Leitfaden der physiologischen Psychologie in 15 Vorlesungen* (7th ed., Jena, 1906), p. 4.

[19] James Rowland Angell, *Psychology* (New York, 1904), p. 1; see also Höffding, *Outlines of Psychology*, p. 12.

reference to a subject or ego, he defines it in terms of content or object. But this conception of consciousness, while avoiding all difficulties in determining the relation of content to ego, suggests no common character through which to unify the various concepts — "sensations, ideas, pains," etc. In spite of the indefiniteness in the conception of consciousness as content plus relation to ego, and in spite of the lack of unity in the conception of it as mere content, most philosophers and psychologists who do not ignore consciousness tend to accept one or the other of these two conceptions. The two conceptions represent two lines of thought which go back the one to Kant and the other to Hume and which resulted from the criticism and the subsequent discarding of the older conception of mind as substance on the part of these two thinkers.

Kant's conception of consciousness is suggested in the "synthetic unity of apperception" as a formal principle of thought and consciousness. It is intended by him primarily as the fundamental principle of all knowledge, but it refers also to the conscious subject — as for instance when he speaks of it as the "I think" which must be such that it can "accompany all my representations," or as the "Vehikel" which "accompanies all categories." [20] This subject or ego is neither a substance nor a will, nor an act or function in time, but rather a pure conscious unity of which all representations, concepts, percepts, volitions, and feelings are content. The value of this concept in defining consciousness was hardly appreciated for three quarters of a century after Kant largely because the faculty psychology of Wolff and Tetens which was accepted by Kant obscured the conception of the subject and its relation to its content. Wundt's "immediate experience," a correction of the theory of mind as "inner sense," reflects the Kantian conception of subject, but it gives the subject a volitional character and allows it to operate in time,[21] thus con-

[20] Immanuel Kant, *Kritik der reinen Vernunft* (2nd ed., Riga, 1787), pp. 136, 406.

[21] Wilhelm Wundt, "Ueber die Definition der Psychologie," *Philosophische Studien* (Leipzig), XII (1896), 12; see also his *Outlines of Psychology*, translated by Charles Judd (New York, 1897), pp. 2–6, 8–9, 13–16.

fusing and missing the full value of the original conception. Calkins's self-psychology might seem at first to fall in line because her definition of psychology as the "science of the self-being-conscious" is suggestive of Kant's "I think." But this similarity is superficial, since she characterizes the self as "relatively persistent," as "complex," as "unique," and as "related to objects" either personal or impersonal,[22] thereby treating the self as a personal rather than as a pure ego. Stout's statement that "psychology is concerned with the relation of what is perceived to the percipient or thinker" [23] involves the conception of a subject, but this, too, falls short, because he defines "psychology as the science of the development of mind " [24] and thus turns to the genetic point of view. Ward has more to offer, yet he too falls short. He refers to a subject or self as more than its presentations. He says "being aware of" as a relation cannot be expressed by one term; we must "admit the necessity of distinguishing between mind or Ego, meaning the unity or continuity of consciousness as a complex of presentations, and Mind or Ego as the subject to which this complex is presented." He says further that the subject of these presentations plus the presentations themselves make up the conception of mind for empirical psychology. He recognizes the relation of "being aware of," as also the "unity" of the mind, though he places this unity on the side of the presentations; but, while distinguishing the subject from the person, he refers to attention as a partial expression of what is meant by consciousness, in this way characterizing consciousness through a special function and treating the subject as performing the act of attending.[25] The distinction between subject and presentation or content and their interrelation are thus not clearly drawn by Ward, so that it is difficult to regard his view as other than a confused statement of Kant's conception. Meinong, too, in distinguishing

[22] Mary Whiton Calkins, *A First Book in Psychology* (New York, 1910), pp. 2–3.

[23] Stout, *A Manual of Psychology*, p. 2.

[24] George Frederick Stout, *Analytic Psychology* (London, 1896), I, 9.

[25] Ward, "Psychology," in *Encyclopaedia Britannica*, XXII, 550–552.

"act" from "content," [26] recognizes something over and above the "content," but he contributes little to the problem as to the nature of "act" and as to the relation of "content" to "act." The points of view of these thinkers — Wundt, Calkins, Stout, Ward, and Meinong — are not truly representative of Kant's conception. They have little in common with him except for the avoidance of defining the subject as substance and the desire to treat the mind as something more than mere content or object.

Kant's "synthetic unity of apperception" suggests two important factors, unity and apperception or consciousness. In other words, this conception includes both unity and consciousness, which may be taken in the sense of awareness or apprehension. It may be convenient here to refer to the two factors as unity and awareness. Many recent thinkers have taken account of one or both of these factors in defining consciousness. Schuppe says, "Absolutely clear, unmistakable, indubitable fact is the I alone," or "the conscious I." [27] This ego he identifies with consciousness as something which can only be "subject." It is not even the "empirical ego" which belongs to the content, nor is it the "individual ego" which is distinguished through content. It is the pure ego and "abstract moment" which is according to Schuppe "not nothing." Then he goes on to say that this ego is absolutely "simple" and is absolutely "point of unity." [28] It is clear that he lays stress upon the unity of consciousness as expressed in the ego, in the subject in contrast with the content. Münsterberg's apprehending consciousness, *vorfindendes Bewusstsein*,[29] in contrast with Schuppe's concept, tends to emphasize awareness. G. E. Moore, too, brings out awareness as a characteristic of mind. He points out that in the experiences of different colors at different times, though the colors are dif-

[26] Alexius Meinong, *Über die Erfahrungsgrundlagen unseres Wissens* (Berlin, 1906), being *Abhandlungen zur Didaktik und Philosophie der Naturwissenschaft*, 1906, Vol. VI, pp. 61–62.

[27] Wilhelm Schuppe, *Erkenntnisstheoretische Logik* (Bonn, 1878), p. 60.

[28] Wilhelm Schuppe, *Grundriss der Erkenntnistheorie und Logik* (Berlin, 1894), pp. 16, 18, 19.

[29] Münsterberg, *Grundzüge der Psychologie*, pp. 202, 209.

ferent, there is something identical in the various experiences. This he calls consciousness [30] or awareness, "the very same unique fact which constitutes every kind of knowledge." [31] Natorp takes account both of awareness and of unity. As his analysis of consciousness goes down to the roots of the problem and is one of the most important contributions on the subject it must here be carefully considered.

Natorp distinguishes three factors in consciousness, the "content," the "I," and the relation between the content and the I. This relation he calls awareness or *Bewusstheit*. The I is aware of the content and the content is for the I, the I and the content being two interrelated terms. But the I is not content or object, nor is it power or activity, it is merely a center or a point of reference for all content. The content may change, but the relation to the I remains the same. Time itself belongs to the content, the I not being in time. The I is thus not appearance, though it is the ground of appearance; and though it is not appearance it can be "verified" and brought out by analysis as something ultimate and irreducible. This conception of consciousness he regards as fundamental to psychology, not in the sense that the I is itself the object to be studied in psychology, but merely that it is the ground of the psychological problem. The problem he defines as the problem of the unity or connection, *Verbindung*, of the content as related to the I in single acts or particular cases of consciousness. This connecting unity is the concrete expression of the relation of the content to the I, as connection in "actual consciousness"; he says it "makes up the object of psychological investigation." [32] Unquestionably Natorp presents in his analysis a conception of the pure ego as a basis of the conception of mind and as the ground of psychological science. The ego is set over against content; it is not in time, it is not will,

[30] George Edward Moore, "The Subject-Matter of Psychology," in *Proceedings of the Aristotelian Society* (London), N.S., X (1910), 39.

[31] George Edward Moore, *Philosophical Studies* (New York, 1922), pp. 27, 29, also pp. 17, 20, 21.

[32] Natorp, *Einleitung in die Psychologie nach kritischer Methode*, pp. 11–15, 23, 26, 27, 30, 32, 36; *Allgemeine Psychologie nach kritischer Methode*, pp. 24, 26–33, 36, 39, 40.

nor is it an individual. Both the factor of awareness and the factor of unity are brought out, and in developing these factors Natorp has carried his analysis beyond that of Kant. It should, however, be noted in regard to the relation of the ego to the content that he regards awareness as more original and fundamental than the connecting unity. He thinks of the I as like the Platonic idea and the connective unity as like that which takes part in the idea, the full significance of the I itself as a kind of all-inclusive unity not being realized in any single phenomenon or connective unity. He is not here trying to suggest an ontological principle in the ego, but merely the relative importance of the ego and the connective unity in defining the psychological problem. His analysis brings out more fully than any other the various factors involved in the Kantian conception.

The subject–object or ego–content theory of consciousness as defined by Natorp has the advantage of being stripped of all non-essentials and brought down to a minimum. Its characteristic feature is to be found in the conception of the ego, the ego as a supertemporal center of reference for all content, as something irreducible and standing in contrast with, but yet related to, content. Without this skeleton of an ego his theory could not stand. Whether there is such an ego making possible consciousness as awareness of content will be taken account of later. The theory of consciousness as merely content must now be considered.

This theory goes back to Hume, who thought of the mind as a flow of perceptions unrelated to any ego. In warding off the conception of the I, he says, "For my part, when I enter most intimately into what I call myself, I always stumble on some particular perception or other, of heat or cold, light or shade, love or hatred, pain or pleasure. I never can catch myself at any time without a perception, and never can observe any thing but the perception." [33] The perceptions make up the content, and the content is for him sufficient. This conception of mind is fundamental to the associationist school

[33] David Hume, *A Treatise of Human Nature*, edited by T. H. Green & T. H. Grose (London, 1874), I, 534.

of psychology, though it is not always carried out consistently. In recent years both Husserl and James have given expression to views similar to that of Hume. In an early work [34] in which he criticizes Natorp's conception of consciousness Husserl says that the existence of the ego cannot be verified, that it cannot be found among the phenomena and therefore is a useless conception in psychology. It is true that in a later work [35] he recognizes the validity of the ego, but in this earlier work he feels that there is a real difficulty in verifying its existence. In *The Principles of Psychology* [36] James has much to say about "the stream of consciousness" and "the passing stream of thought." This "stream" is for him essentially content. In criticizing the Kantian conception of "the pure ego" he regards this ego as a sort of remnant of the old substantial ego and he says of it that it is "simply nothing; as ineffectual and windy an abortion as Philosophy can show." Also, in distinguishing between the "me" and the "I" he does not intend the "I" to suggest the pure ego. By the "me" he means "the empirical person" and by the "I" "the judging Thought," both belonging to the content of consciousness. In an essay called "Does Consciousness Exist?" [37] he even questions the value of the conception of consciousness, particularly as this term has tended to refer to entities, to souls, and to egos. He believes that the only value in the conception of consciousness lies in its reference to the function of knowledge, and knowledge, he believes, can be explained through the relation of one part of "pure experience" to another part, in other words, all in terms of content. Holt's conception of the "neutral cross-section" [38] also leaves out of account any ego and makes consciousness purely a matter of content. Other adherents of the Humean view need not be mentioned, but it should be

[34] Edmund Husserl, *Logische Untersuchungen* (Halle, 1900–01), II, 340–344.

[35] Edmund Husserl, "Ideen zu einer reinen Phänomenologie und phänomenologischen Philosophie," in *Jahrbuch für Philosophie und phänomenologische Forschung*, I (Halle, 1913), 86.

[36] William James, *The Principles of Psychology* (New York, 1890), I, 329–373.

[37] William James, *Essays in Radical Empiricism* (New York, 1912), pp. 1–38.

[38] Holt, *The Concept of Consciousness*, pp. 166–207.

noted that in recent years many thinkers have turned toward this theory and away from all conceptions of the pure ego.

The content theory has undoubtedly resulted from a process of elimination. The old soul-substance became the Kantian "I think," with Natorp and others a mere skeleton of an ego, finally to be dropped by such thinkers as James, Husserl, and Holt. Hume, of course, did suggest the theory before Kant, but it is only in recent years that it has been seriously opposed to the Kantian theory in psychological discussion. It avoids all difficulties with regard to determining the nature and existence of the pure ego and it attempts to explain all the legitimate demands of a knower out of the content which can be found; in fact it recognizes only that which can be found and regards the finder as belonging among the things to be found. It simplifies the conception of consciousness, but the question may be raised as to whether it does not oversimplify it. The unity of consciousness has become the "unity of the passing moment" and mind is to be thought of as essentially temporal. According to this theory, time rather than ego may well stand out as fundamental to consciousness.

In the discussion of the conception of psychology as a science of the individual or of the relation of experience to the individual it was said that the individual might be defined either on the basis of the mind or on the basis of the body. If based on the conception of the mind it led to the conception of consciousness and to a psychology independent of physical science. If based on the conception of the body it tended to make psychology a branch of biology and led ultimately to behaviorism. In the ego–content theory the individual might be identified with the ego or with some part of the content or with both the ego and the content, while in the content theory it is connected with some part or phase of the content. Where the individual is defined on the basis of the body, the body is considered as fundamental in the explanation of mental phenomena. Greater emphasis may then be laid on the body so that in behaviorism the original mental phenomena tend to be neglected or even to be regarded as non-existent.

Instead of referring to the relation of experience to the individual or to the individual with its experiences, the behaviorist refers to the relation of the organism to its environment. But the transition from the older view of mental phenomena to the behavioristic view was a gradual one. From the days of Hume and Kant down to the latter part of the nineteenth century the psychologist was interested in the structure and composition of mental phenomena, in "states of consciousness." With the growing emphasis upon mental process and function it became increasingly difficult to give an account of mental phenomena without reference to the organism. An explanation of perception, habit, instinct, emotion, association, will, and even thought itself was found to be intimately bound up with the activity of the nervous system. Angell appreciated this difficulty when he said: "In our study of mental processes we shall adopt the biological point of view just now dominant in psychology, and regard consciousness, not as a metaphysical entity to be investigated apart from other things, but rather as one among many manifestations of organic life, to be understood properly only when regarded in connection with life phenomena." He laid it down as a postulate that "the real human organism is a psychophysical organism," holding that "all the operations of consciousness — all our sensations, all our emotions, and all our acts of will — . . . [are] so many expressions of organic adaptations to our environment." [39]

This point of view may be referred to as that of functionalism. It was not the intention of the functionalist to give up the conception of the psychophysical individual or organism; he intended to give a better foundation to and a fuller explanation of mental phenomena by linking the mind to the body, not to discard the psychical for the physical organism. But the swing toward biology was not to be stopped. The definiteness of the physical organism, the unity of the nervous

[39] Angell, *Psychology*, pp. 6, 7; see also James, *The Principles of Psychology*, I, 128–144.

system, and the less complicated method of explanation in physical terms only led certain psychologists to make psychology a branch of biology by treating all matters psychological as phases of the reaction of organism to environment. Undoubtedly the study of animal psychology, in which only animal behavior but not mental process can be observed directly, helped to bring about the behavioristic point of view. Thus the tendency away from a static psychology toward a psychology which emphasized processes and functions led to behaviorism. Meyer [40] and Watson [41] were among the first to give full expression to this conception of psychology.[42]

Watson speaks as follows: "Psychology as the behaviorist views it is a purely objective experimental branch of natural science." It has no more need of "introspection" than have "chemistry and physics." "The behavior of man and the behavior of animals must be considered" as "on the same plane." "Consciousness in a psychological sense" can be dispensed with, though it may possibly be regarded as the "instrument or tool with which all scientists work." [43] Furthermore, "introspection" is "a serious bar to progress," and "states of consciousness" not being "objectively verifiable" can never become "data for science." In fact, "the behaviorist finds no evidence for mental existences or mental processes of any kind." [44] Believing consciousness to be neither "a definite nor a usable concept," behaviorism holds that psychology is the science of the "behavior of the human being" or organism. It is thus "a natural science that takes the whole field of human adjustments as its own." "It is different from physiology only in the grouping of its problems, not in fundamentals or in central viewpoint." [45]

[40] Max Friedrich Meyer, *The Fundamental Laws of Human Behavior* (Boston, 1911).

[41] John Broadus Watson, *Behavior, An Introduction to Comparative Psychology* (New York, 1914).

[42] Jared Sparks Moore, *The Foundations of Psychology* (Princeton, 1921), pp. 27–65; Walter Bowers Pillsbury, *The History of Psychology* (New York, 1929), pp. 271–299.

[43] Watson, *Behavior*, pp. 1, 27.

[44] John Broadus Watson, *Psychology, from the Standpoint of a Behaviorist* (Philadelphia and London, 1919), pp. 1–2.

[45] John Broadus Watson, *Behaviorism* (New York, 1925), pp. 2, 11.

As characterized by Watson, psychology is properly the study of the behavior of organisms. As a psychological theory it stands at the opposite pole from the ego–content theory. Mind is essentially behavior or the ways in which an organism reacts to its environment. To know the mind it is only necessary to observe the behavior of the organism, and to have scientific or accurate knowledge of mind it is only necessary to study the laws and conditions of behavior. Undoubtedly one of the great advantages of behaviorism is to be found in this attempt to treat mind as having a place in the space–time system, to regard psychology as a branch of biology and therefore as a branch of physical science, and in so doing to use the methods of observation and experiment as used by the natural sciences. In thus keeping clear of consciousness and so avoiding the method of introspection, behaviorism gives unity to the conception of the mind and defines with greater definiteness the line of research for psychology. To attain this unity and definiteness it leaves much out of account which has generally been considered mental and psychological. In substituting behavior for consciousness it has entirely changed the character of psychology. Though in attaining its ideal it has sacrificed many cherished conceptions, it has been consistent in trying to limit psychology to one sphere of knowledge, to the field of biological science.

The result of the foregoing attempt to characterize the various conceptions of mind and definitions of psychology may be stated briefly as follows:

1. Psychology is a science of the real and not of the ideal. As concerned with the mind as something real or factual it is opposed to the normative sciences of ethics and aesthetics as sciences of norms or ideals. Though the real object of psychology and the ideal objects of the normative sciences may be in some way related, the primary interest of these sciences is essentially different.

2. Psychology as a science of the real is also distinguished from logic as the science of the fundamental relations, laws, or norms of all truth whether of the real or of the ideal. In spite of some confusion of logic with psychology, logic can

never be regarded as a branch of psychology or as subordinate to it.

3. Psychology as a science of one phase or part of the real is distinguished from ontology as the study of ultimate reality, taken as a whole. Although according to some schools of thought mind is suggestive of the character of ultimate reality, psychology is not concerned with the final framework of things.

4. Among the sciences of the real, psychology is usually opposed to physical science. The mind is taken to be an inner as opposed to an outer reality. It is said to be in time but not in space, whereas the physical world is both in space and in time. This conception is unsatisfactory because it is difficult to conceive of a temporal reality which is not spatial and because the attempted separation of the mind from the physical world is not possible without some further conception over and above that of time.

5. Psychology is sometimes defined as the science of the individual as opposed to the over-individual, or as the science of any truth, reality, or object as related to the individual. This definition is important in calling attention to the particular or concrete character of the mind but it is ambiguous unless it further defines the individual, as the individual may be associated either with consciousness or with the body.

6. According to one view, psychology is essentially the science of consciousness and the mind is thought to be defined by that conception. There are two theories as to the fundamental nature of consciousness, the ego–content theory and the content theory.

7. According to the ego–content theory, mind implies an ego standing in relation to a content or a subject conscious of an object. The relation between the ego and the content may be expressed as a knower knowing the known or as an experiencer experiencing the experienced. The ego may be thought of as a point of reference for the content, or as a unity of the content, and again it may be thought of as an awareness of the content. Unity and awareness would seem to

be essential features of the relation. Some thinkers regard the ego or subject as also a will or self, but the will and the self are not included in the ego in the original Kantian conception, and as they can both be included under the content it only complicates and obscures the conception of the ego to add them to it. Some thinkers also regard the ego as well as the content as in time. This again leads to difficulties, as it would tend to make the ego content, and time itself would not be related to the ego as content. If the ego is to be that to which all content is related, it must be supertemporal. This theory is essentially that of a supertemporal ego which both unites and is aware of content however diverse.

8. According to the content theory, mind is only content, object, or experience. All unity, awareness, knowledge, etc., are explained on the basis of relations belonging to the content. The mind is therefore in time, and its unity is the unity of the present or momentary content, the shifting groupings of content making up the mind. The inclusion of the content in time may easily suggest its reference to space and therefore seem to include mind in the physical world, but this theory treats mind as consciousness, or as experience, or in Hume's language as "perception," rather than as a physical or bodily function.

9. According to another theory, psychology is not concerned with consciousness but is rather the science of the behavior of organisms. This theory, known as behaviorism, was the result of an attempt to explain conscious functions by reference to the nervous system. This reference to the nervous system for purposes of explanation increased the importance of the brain. The center of interest then easily passed from consciousness to the nervous system, and the mind was finally thought to be made up of the reactions of the nervous system to the organism's environment. The nervous system and its behavior as compared with consciousness are more accessible and also determinable according to the methods of natural science. This theory thus makes psychology a branch of biology.

In this statement three rather extreme theories of mind stand out, three theories which contrast rather sharply with one another: the ego–content theory, the content theory, and behaviorism. Many intermediate and less radical theories there are, but these three theories represent the logical conclusions of certain very definite tendencies in psychology and philosophy. They are tendencies which cannot be neglected in any consideration of the nature of mind. In the evaluation of these theories the relation of psychology to the other sciences and the distinction of mind from the other objects of knowledge must be borne in mind, as also the conception of mind as in some sense individual or concrete.

Before any criticism of these theories is offered some account of the general methods of psychology should be given.

In common with other sciences, particularly the physical sciences, psychology may be said to depend upon the methods of description and explanation. To describe is to fix and define facts by bringing them under class concepts, and to explain is to place these facts in or assign them to the settings or systems to which they belong. Description runs to detail while explanation takes account of the larger connections. Three kinds of description stand out in psychology as of fundamental importance; they are description by introspection, by external observation, and by reconstruction.

Introspection is internal observation or the direct observation of the mind by the mind itself. Consciousness is brought to bear upon itself, and any description based upon any such internal observation is first-hand description. "Introspective observation," "looking into our own minds," says James, is "what we have to rely on first and foremost and always." [46] In fact, most psychologists have regarded this method as the primary method of psychology and as peculiar to it. Structuralists, functionalists, *Gestalt* psychologists, self-psychologists, have all depended upon introspection. The behaviorists only have tried to avoid it. As they either neglect consciousness or do not accept it as a fact they have little use for a method

[46] James, *The Principles of Psychology*, I, 185; see also Stout, *A Manual of Psychology*, p. 14.

of observing it. This method may therefore be said to be a method appropriate to all psychology which connects mind with consciousness. It must be taken account of then in criticizing the ego–content and the content theories of mind.

External observation is the observation of the activities and reactions of the organism as signs of mind and mental activity. It is based upon the assumption that bodily activity accompanies mental activity or is itself mental activity. For the psychologist who holds that mind is primarily consciousness, this kind of observation is of value mainly as a supplement to introspection. Having observed conscious facts by introspection and having noted corresponding bodily activities, such as facial movements or contractions of the muscles, he may be able to detect the presence of certain mental activities by merely observing the activities of the organism. Perry [47] goes so far as to make external observation an independent source of knowledge of mind; but without some basis of knowledge in introspection external observation would seem to be of little help. An animal's mind must be studied mainly on the basis of external observation, although without some idea of human minds based on introspection it would be difficult to describe the animal's mind. For the behaviorist external observation is the only proper method, because for him mind is the behavior of organisms and such behavior can only be described on the basis of direct observation of the organisms. One advantage may be claimed by this kind of observation over introspection. In introspection one mind can only be observed by one individual, namely by that individual mind itself, whereas in external observation one organism may be observed by many individuals, the chances of error in observation thus being minimized. Also, it should be noted that external observation is the kind of observation very generally used in physical science, and that therefore those who hope to make psychology a branch of physical science will naturally turn to this kind of observation as fundamental.

[47] Ralph Barton Perry, *Present Philosophical Tendencies* (New York, 1912), pp. 286–305.

Description by reconstruction is a construction or reconstruction of the mind, of its structure and functions, of its unity and composition, by using the content present in consciousness as a basis for or a suggestion or sign of a content not present or no longer present in consciousness or, if in consciousness, not easily observed. Introspection easily becomes recollection or retrospection because the immediate content under observation quickly passes into the past and can only be observed or studied in memory. So long as the interest lies in determining the nature of the structure and functions of content, which, though it has been present, has slipped into the past, the method may still be regarded as that of introspection; but as soon as the interest becomes an interest in determining the nature of the past by putting that which is past together again as it was in the original experience, then the method becomes one of reconstruction. In other words, introspection may include both memory and direct observation, but any further hypothetical construction of the mind would fall under reconstruction. Again, if the constitution of a state is studied with a view to understanding the workings of the mind or minds of those who composed the constitution, or if a work of art is studied in order to understand the composition of the mind of the artist, mind is studied and described by reconstruction. An animal's mind may be reconstructed out of elements in the content of the human mind, or the texture of the human mind in its earlier stages before the beginning of civilization may be constructed or reconstructed by subtraction from certain phases of the human mind as it is today. A more definite method of reconstruction is developed by Natorp.[48] He holds that the objective sciences come first, and that after the objectifications and constructions of those sciences have been made, subjective science, that is, the determination of mind, or consciousness, or immediate experience, may be made by reconstruction of the factors brought out in the objective constructions. He believes that the mind objectifies, and that by a study of its

[48] Natorp, *Einleitung in die Psychologie nach kritischer Methode*, pp. 88–118; *Allgemeine Psychologie nach kritischer Methode*, pp. 189–213.

objectifications, the original source of these objectifications, the mind, can be understood. The object leads away from the mind, so that to get at the mind it is necessary to move back from the object to the subject or mind. Objectifications in space–time, space–time itself as an object, moral systems, aesthetic objects, or any purely logical relations, may serve as the objective basis for such reconstruction. It should be pointed out here that reconstruction is an independent method and not to be identified with introspection or external observation, though psychologists generally have not paid much attention to it. As a descriptive method it is more hypothetical than the other two methods, but it is a necessary method if psychological description and the general scope of psychology are not to be narrowed down to that which can be directly observed. Furthermore, mind or consciousness as immediate experience cannot be fully determined without the help of this less direct method. More will be said about it later.

The three methods of description are all used by most psychologists, but the relative importance of these methods and the emphasis laid upon one or another of them vary very much with the various conceptions of psychology. The behaviorists emphasize the method of external observation — indeed, they claim it to be the only proper psychological method — though in fact they do at times use the other two methods. Those who accept the content theory of mind would in most cases regard introspection as the primary method, although they would recognize the other two methods, particularly the method of external observation, as supplementary but of no value apart from introspection. For them mind centers in consciousness, and though consciousness includes only content, the direct observation of that content is basic. The followers of the ego–content theory ought to regard and in some cases do regard the method of reconstruction as fundamental. Because of the emphasis on consciousness they tend to put introspection first and to make the other two methods quite secondary. Yet however valuable introspection and external observation may be, the method appropriate to the conception of mind carried out by the ego–content theory is the method of reconstruction. This method increases in importance as the ego–content theory becomes more consistent. Certain phases of that theory of consciousness make introspection insufficient and involve the broader and more complicated method of reconstruction.

As for explanation, if it means the reference of facts to their proper settings or systems, then there must be as many kinds of explanation as there are possible systems of truth. But in natural science the term explanation usually means causal explanation, that is, fitting the fact into its proper place in the causal nexus in space–time by determining what its conditions or causes are in that nexus. As this kind of explanation holds such an important place in knowledge, and as it must be distinguished from other kinds of explanation, it might be convenient to use the terms causal explanation and non-causal explanation. Reference of an act of will to its place in the moral order or reduction of a proposition in geometry to the postulates of the geometrical system to which it belongs would be examples of non-causal explanation. In psychology little has been said about non-causal explanation. In behaviorism causal explanation would naturally hold; and in the content theory of consciousness, inasmuch as the content is in time, explanation is generally assumed to be causal. In the ego–content theory, however, non-causal explanation may be required, particularly so far as the ego and the nontemporal relation of the content to the ego are involved. Probably this theory offers more dimensions of explanation than the other two theories.

With due consideration for what has now been said in regard to the methods of description and explanation and in regard to their relation to the three fundamental theories of mind, the criticism of those theories can be undertaken.

First, as to behaviorism. Though many may regard this theory as extreme it should not be forgotten that it has attempted to bring psychology into the fold of the natural or physical sciences. It finds the unity of the mind in the brain, and it regards the individual as the concrete physical individual whose functions can be investigated by the usual methods of natural science. As these functions take place in space and time they are not explained by any reference to non-causal systems but as having their place in the causal nexus in space–time. Thus by falling back upon the description of and experimentation with the functions of the organism as unified in the nervous system, and by using the method of causal explanation, behaviorism, as was said above, makes psychology a branch of biology. In this way psychology is thought to take its place as a genuine science and no longer as a discipline claiming special privileges. Yet by giving greater unity, definiteness, and consistency to the problem of psychology, and by making the mind more concrete and accessible, it may have lost sight of much which is properly mental and which lies within the scope of psychology. Just as a melody may be conceived of as having a definite rhythmic pattern and as still having many other values, so the mind may well stand in relation to the functions of the nervous system and at the same time stand in other equally important relations. Sensations or associations can be referred to activities of the brain but they can also be sensed or felt, that is, they can be phases or functions of consciousness; and consciousness can hardly be identified with brain function although it may stand in very intimate relation to such function. Still, in spite of the claim on behalf of mind as inclusive of consciousness over and above brain function, behaviorism has pushed consciousness off the scientific stage, and it has done this largely because it does not regard consciousness as a proper scientific object or conception. But although consciousness seems vague and inaccessible, if it can be conceived of at all, it is an object of knowledge and therefore of science, though possibly not of physical science. That it is not conceived of as a function in space–time does not prevent it from having a place in knowledge and being determined by an appropriate method. Therefore, when behaviorism tries to strengthen psychology by making it a part of biology it drops out a field of knowledge which may rightly be considered psychological. It sees only one side of the picture; it clarifies one part of the field by leaving other parts out of account.

Though it may be difficult to convince the behaviorists of the scientific value of consciousness, or even of its existence, the question may arise as to which of the two conceptions, consciousness or nerve-function, stands closer to what is meant by the mental or psychical. Should the results of the research done by behaviorists and others in the study of the reactions of the organism to the environment as unified through the unity of the nervous system be regarded as the substance of psychology? In other words, should the study of reflexes, instincts, habits, emotions, language, etc., as forms of the reaction to the environment, be called psychology? Or should the study of consciousness, including the great variety of detail brought to light through introspection and reconstruction, be known as psychological investigation or psychology? To call knowledge of consciousness psychology is more in keeping with ordinary thought as well as with the history of thought. It might be possible to distinguish between two kinds of psychology, biological psychology and the psychology of consciousness, but since biological psychology can be classed as biology, it would seem better to reserve the term psychology to cover the psychology of consciousness. In any case, in this work the term psychology will be so used. There is here of course no intention to minimize the value of the research done by behaviorists, nor to neglect an important point of view brought out by behaviorism.

Secondly, the content theory. If the behavioristic theory neglects consciousness, the content theory is centered in it. It is interested primarily in the content of consciousness, whether it conceives of that content as making up personal history or as merely the content of the passing moment. It is concerned with the original content or phenomena of consciousness, with percepts, images, concepts, volitions, feeling, etc., as they appear and are determined by introspection. It may not be averse to an explanation of these phenomena by reference to functions of the brain, but it does regard them as the primary data of mind and as not identical with brain function. It advocates a psychology which does not set aside direct and immediate experience. But now it should be pointed out that while this theory recognizes consciousness, or what may well be called mental phenomena, it stands in unstable equilibrium. On the one hand, as the phenomena of consciousness are in time and are therefore in flux and subject to change, they may be said to be made up of processes and functions; and as the processes and functions may best be understood in connection with the processes and functions of the brain, the phenomena may be more naturally regarded as processes and functions of the organism. Or to state the matter in a more general way, if the mental phenomena are in time they are also in space, since, as was explained above, temporal but non-spatial phenomena are not conceivable; and if the phenomena are in both space and time they are physical phenomena. On the other hand, if the phenomena are to be regarded as not exclusively physical phenomena they must stand in relation to something which is not spatio-temporal. If consciousness is regarded as more than content, that is, as implying reference to a conscious unity or to awareness, then it may be possible to save the phenomena from becoming merely physical; but in that case the content theory will have to be given up in favor of the ego–content theory. Thus the content theory cannot stand on its own feet. It must either relegate mental phenomena to physical science and explain the content of consciousness as functions of the organism in space–time, or it must add to its conception of content some such conception as that of the ego, to which the content is related, something to prevent the content from being merely a space-time phenomenon.

Mind not being adequately conceived of by behaviorism and not being sufficiently distinguished from things physical by the content theory, the ego–content theory must be examined with great care. This theory defines mind as consciousness; therefore a careful analysis of consciousness becomes necessary. The theory is an old one and regarded by many as vague, but if mind is not to become merely an organic function or a phenomenon in the causal nexus in space–time, the essential features of this theory should be brought out as clearly as possible with the view to supplementing the other two theories.

The ego–content theory as distinct from the content theory holds that over and above the content there is an ego. This ego is not a self or a person, nor is it a substantial entity contrasted with the content. It is introduced rather to show that mind cannot be expressed merely as content but must include consciousness of content, and consciousness of content seems to include besides content two important features, namely unity and awareness. It would be more accurate to say of this theory of mind that it means to include the factors of unity, awareness, content, and their interrelations. To make this clear consciousness may be characterized as involving the following features:

1. Unity. Consciousness is a unity, though not a *bare* unity nor a unity *in the manifold or among* the contents which it unifies, but rather a unity or connection *of* the manifold or content, a union of this content in one whole or one group.

2. Awareness. Consciousness is awareness, a being aware of something, its content. It is not awareness on the part of one part of the content of some other part of the content. It cannot be easily defined, but is suggested by the relations of knowing, experiencing, feeling, and other similar relations. As a relation it seems to imply not only content of which there is awareness but also an ego which is aware. The full relation with its terms might be expressed as ego being aware of content. The ego can be referred to only as a term implied by awareness but not as further determinable.

3. Content. Consciousness is also content. Though unity and awareness imply content, and there could be no unity and awareness without it, they do not in general define the content. The content is a manifold made up of a vast variety of relations; the psychologists usually refer to it as made up of sensations, percepts, images, concepts, volitions, feelings, etc. Temporal and spatial relations as well as all features which make up the self are included in the content.

4. Limitation of content. The content of which there is unity and awareness is limited, that is, as related to unity and

awareness the factors making up the detail of the content are finite in number.

The unity (1) of consciousness as here defined is not an abstract unity off by itself, nor is it an item or relation on the side of the content. Furthermore it is not a container of the content, something in which the content floats, and it does not define the nature of the content. It would be more correct to conceive of it as a relation of which the factors in the content are the terms. This relation may be thought of as a unifying or grouping of the manifold factors of the content, as a binding or holding together of that manifold. The content may be very varied in character and in its interrelations, and it may constantly be undergoing change. The manifold of the content may be as compact and continuous as the various factors in a field of color, or it may be as separate and discrete as a tone, a color, and a feeling of pleasure, yet this manifold will fall within the group or whole of the conscious unity. Any part of the content may form a group or unity, but the group or unity here meant is the unity of all the content. The unity of consciousness, even when defined as a grouping of content, may seem unimportant and arbitrary, and it may seem to be little more than the sum or the whole of the content, but its full significance will appear after awareness has been considered.

Awareness (2) is a most difficult feature to characterize. Since it is always present as a feature of consciousness, and unlike unity has nothing analogous to it on the side of the content, it easily escapes notice, and can be gotten at only indirectly. Awareness suggests immediate or direct consciousness of something. Immediate experience of a percept or image, direct knowledge of a concept or object, an appearance appearing or being given to an ego, and feeling a feeling, are various ways of stating the relation of awareness. The immediacy here involved is not the relation of a content to some further content, or a part of the content to some other part — that is, it is not knowledge as the assimilation of new to old knowledge or the subsumption of particulars under a universal, no matter how direct or close the assimilation and subsumption may be. Such knowledge could involve awareness only if it were present to or given to an ego, only if there were actual consciousness of it. The organization of knowledge belongs to the content, whereas the relation of awareness can only be brought out by contrast with the content. As contrasted with the content, awareness seems to involve two matters, the nature of the relation of awareness itself and the significance of the ego which seems to be implied in it. These two matters must now be considered.

The relation of awareness may be suggested in various ways though it cannot easily be brought into the light of day. Consider for instance a one-cell organism. If it shows signs of being psychical as well as physical it might possibly be thought to have the feeling of pleasure when absorbing nourishment. If it has such a feeling it would hardly be sufficient to regard that feeling as merely the quale pleasure. Beside the feeling as the quale the feeling would also be felt. The feeling would thus imply two factors, the quale pleasure and some sort of awareness of it. This dual character of feeling stands out in contrast with the character of physical objects, which seem to involve no such duality. As attributing feeling to a one-cell organism is based upon reconstruction of features taken from the human mind, a closer approach to awareness may be made by considering the human mind itself. As was stated earlier in this chapter, in the experiences of different colors at different times there is, according to G. E. Moore, something identical connected with the different experiences, and this something, which is a "unique fact" in all knowledge, he regards as the feature which is called awareness. Here awareness is characterized as a feature of all knowledge and all experience, but just because it is a universal feature of consciousness and is always present it is difficult to distinguish it and to discover its character. It might be thought that this general feature of mind could be brought to light just as the general feature of time is determined. Though time as a general feature may be easily overlooked or forgotten, it can be brought out as the form of change or alteration of content. But as an alteration of content it is a phase of content while awareness is not. As a feature of consciousness it always stands over against content, being neither a general feature of all the factors of consciousness applying to each factor separately nor a relation *in* the content holding between any of those factors. Furthermore, not only is awareness not content, but it cannot be observed directly or brought to light in its full significance by any simple procedure. In spite of the suggestions that feeling implies awareness and that some such "unique fact" such as awareness is involved in knowledge or consciousness, it might seem that psychology would have to give up the conception of awareness, because its very universality makes it useless, and because the fact that it must be distinguished from content and cannot be directly observed makes it inaccessible. Shall it be regarded, then, as something indefinable and unverifiable, as a possible hypothesis but as one which has nothing to offer in definition of the mind?

Though awareness cannot be verified from within, that is, by an examination of consciousness, it can at least be made clear that there is such a factor as awareness by a comparison of consciousness with truth and reality beyond it. It might possibly be thought, because awareness is said to be a feature of all experience and consciousness, that it is also a character accompanying all relations and all phases of truth and reality. But it may easily be shown that the content of consciousness implies, though it does not include, relations and phases of truth of which there is no awareness. For instance, a man walking by an unoccupied house which has long been closed may know that the house contains furniture and objects but neither he nor any other conscious being may know the exact arrangement or configuration of such furniture and objects. Something escapes awareness, so that it cannot be regarded as a universal character of things and always conjoined with them. But awareness may be that feature of consciousness by means of which the content of consciousness and that which lies beyond are differentiated. It may well be referred to as a kind of "light" of consciousness. As an object on which light is thrown stands out in contrast with objects not illuminated, so awareness of content may be brought out when reference is made to something of which there is no awareness. If, then, awareness cannot be verified by direct observation, it can be verified as a fact of consciousness by the indirect method just explained.

The result of the foregoing attempt to define awareness is that it has been possible to verify the fact that there is awareness, but not to make clear what its actual nature is. Not only is it contrasted with relations beyond consciousness and yet considered universal to consciousness, but it is also said to imply an ego. The ego is usually regarded as standing in relation of awareness to the content of consciousness, that is, the ego is treated as aware of content. The ego and the content are then the terms of the relation of awareness which connects them in one direction only, from ego to content. The direction might be reversed by stating the relation as that of the content given to the ego, in which case the direction of the relation would be from the content to the ego. Now it might seem that by this introduction of the ego the concept of awareness might be made explicit. Unfortunately, however, the ego is just as difficult to characterize as awareness. It should not be forgotten that the ego here intended is not the empirical ego, nor the ego as will, nor in any sense an ego in time. It is merely an ego implied by the relation of awareness. It can at best be assumed to be nothing more than a term or terminal of that relation and internal to it. The value of such an ego seems to be only formal, but before any conclusion in regard to it is drawn it should be considered in connection with the concept of the unity of consciousness.

In the ego–content theory, the ego is not only thought to be aware of the content, but it is also thought to unify the content. It is related to the content by both unity and awareness. It unifies in being aware of content and it is aware of content in unifying. It should further be made clear that not only are unity and awareness relations or features of a relation of ego to content, but each involves the other. The unity is determined by awareness of content; that which the ego unifies may be defined as that — its content — of which it is aware as distinguished from that of which it is not aware; and awareness in turn is unified awareness of content — that is, the ego in being aware of its content is not aware of the different parts of the content separately but in unity. In other words, there is unified awareness or awareness-unity of content, and whichever phase of the relation is emphasized the ego is supposed to perform both the functions of unifying and of being aware.

In the attempt to determine the character of the relations of unity and of awareness it would seem to have been a mistake to introduce the conception of an ego. If so, the ego–content theory needs to be revised. Because men prefer terms to relations and think terminally more easily than relationally, it is natural in analyzing consciousness to emphasize the ego and the content as important terms, and then to add unity or awareness as relations holding between those terms. Now in any analysis it is important to determine which relations are the primary or original ones before any consideration is given to those which are secondary and derivative. The object of analysis is to clarify the fundamental synthesis. In the relation *aRb*, *R* relates the terms *a* and *b* or expresses the relation of the term *a* to the term *b*, and in the example *the hammer hits the nail, hitting* is a relation of the term *hammer* to the term *nail*. The relation *R*, or the relation *hitting*, connects its terms and connects them in a specific way. If these relations are regarded as primary relations or original syntheses there are certain other relations which may be regarded as secondary or derivative and dependent on the primary relations. The relations of *a* to *R*, *R* to *b*, the *hammer* to *hitting*, and *hitting* to the *nail* are such secondary or dependent relations. But to regard the relation of *a* to *R* and of *R* to *b* as expressing in a more profound way the relation *aRb* would be a serious mistake. With the relation of *the hammer hitting the nail* further secondary relations might be mentioned. If the *hitting* is contrasted with the *hammer* and the *nail*, instead of being regarded as being related to the *hammer* and *nail*, the *hitting* itself might be regarded as the relation between the *carpenter* on the one hand and the *hammer* and *nail* on the other. Or the *carpenter* might be combined with the *hitting*, the function which he performs, and then further related to the *hammer* and the *nail*. Yet these secondary relations remain secondary relations and should not be confounded with primary relations. In the same way unity and awareness are not usually treated as primary relations. Either the ego like the carpenter is said to perform the function of unifying and being aware of the content, or unity and awareness are treated as a kind of center or ego, and then like the relations of the *a* to the *R* and the *R* to the *b* they are treated as a term related to the content. In neither case are the primary relations of unity and awareness brought out, namely as relations *of* the content though not themselves content, the content making up only the terms of the relations. The view held here is that unity and awarenesss are relations or possibly a part of a group of relations relating and connecting the content but not as part of the content. They may be thought of as supertemporal or superphenomenal relations. But there is no need of making an ego out of them or of making them imply an ego as an ultimate term. It may be possible to verify the fact that there is unity and the fact that there is awareness, but to imply an ego means to go beyond the two primary relations. The ego–content theory is misleading, and if the foregoing analysis is accurate the ego should be eliminated or at least not regarded as essential or of prime importance to an analysis of consciousness. It would then seem wiser to refer to the theory not as the ego–content theory but as the awareness-unity theory.

This modification of the ego–content theory with the ego either left out or pushed into the background might seem to lead back to the content theory of consciousness. Unity and awareness might appear to be in danger of being submerged in the content. But as long as unity and awareness are intended as relations to which the content supplies the terms they cannot themselves become content without becoming terms and thereby losing their status as relations relating the content or terms. The awareness-unity theory is therefore in no danger of being identified with a mere content theory.

Should it furthermore seem that awareness is unanalyzable and consequently negligible it should be pointed out that in the tone *A* or in the taste *sweet* there is a quality which is unanalyzable but which is nevertheless taken account of in psychology. And should it be said that unity is a purely formal relation it should not be forgotten that unity goes with awareness and that awareness may be sufficient to differentiate an awareness-unity from other unities.

It may well be that unity and awareness represent respectively the quantitative and qualitative sides of the superphenomenal or supercontent relations of consciousness. Unity may stand for the grouping of the manifold in the content which is defined by awareness of the manifold, and awareness may stand for a general character or relation under which the manifold falls in the unity. It might also be true that unity and awareness express two sides of a relational system which apart from content constitutes consciousness. But reflections such as these lead to ontology. Further considerations of the ego–content theory, or rather of the awareness-unity theory, must now lead to a consideration of the content and its limitation.

The content (3) of consciousness, though implied by awareness-unity, is so implied only in the sense that relations imply terms, not in the sense that the relations define the terms. In fact the content may be what it will so long as there is content, and since the content seems to be defined and determined independently of awareness-unity, the awareness-unity may be said to be an external relation, a non-implicative relation of the content; that is, no content implies that it must stand in the awareness-unity relation or as a term in that relation. Not only is this relation external to the content, but the content is a manifold involving relations beyond the content and not within the awareness-unity relation. Besides, the content is constantly changing, and this flowing character of the content should never be regarded as a kind of relation between the content and awareness-unity but always as a phase of the content. The awareness-unity relation is not itself in time, for if it were a relation in time there could be no awareness or consciousness of time. Furthermore, the consciousness of supertemporal relations of teleological conceptions and of the structure of truth could not easily be understood if the awareness-unity were limited in time. Perhaps the identification of time and change with content can best be expressed by the statement that consciousness is not in time but that time is in consciousness. Then it should also be noted that volition or will and the self are phases of the content and should not be confused in any way with the awareness-unity or any ego assumed to be implied in that relation. Marshall's [49] suggestion of a "clear and distinct" "presentation" or content over against a "vague and elusive" "background" or "Self" is not satisfactory, because such a background or Self, though vague, is part of the content and is also no true substitute for the awareness-unity relation. To put it briefly, the content, while standing in the awareness-unity relation, is determined largely independently of the awareness-unity, and it includes time, change, will, and self as well as supertemporal relations.

The limitation (4) of content in the awareness-unity relation has never been treated as of equal importance with unity, awareness, or content, and it may seem to many to be a secondary matter. But without the inclusion of the limitation of content as a fundamental feature of the awareness-unity theory, this theory would be of little value in the definition of mind. There is no difficulty in making clear that such limitation is a fact. Höfler [50] refers in a general way to this limitation or narrowness, *Enge*, of consciousness, and Baldwin [51] mentions it in his discussion of the "area" of consciousness. More specifically it may be said that in the "area" of consciousness the number of sense data, the number of factors in an image, the number of concepts which can be brought together in judgment or thought, the variety of features in a purpose, and these all taken together, are always

[49] Henry Rutgers Marshall, *Consciousness* (New York, 1909), p. 4.

[50] Höfler, *Psychologie*, p. 13.

[51] James Mark Baldwin, *Handbook of Psychology, Senses and Intellect* (2nd ed., New York, 1890), pp. 63–64.

finite in number. "Always" might seem to mean that the number of factors of the content are at all times and therefore at any one time limited. However true this may be, and however it may be that the time-span in time perception offers a good example of the limitation of content, no phase of time should be used in characterizing this limitation. The only accurate way to define it is to refer the content to awareness-unity, that is, to regard the content of which there is unity and awareness as finite. And not only must the area of which there is unity and awareness be conceived of as being limited by having a sort of edge, but, as much of the detail of the content cannot be further analyzed, its structure must also be thought of as limited. For instance, sensations and feelings include factors or units which cannot be broken up. Should it be thought that concepts include unlimited factors, it should be remembered that they do so only by implication of relations which lie outside the awareness-unity relation. In a proposition in which the factor *m* is meant to repeat itself *ad infinitum*, only a limited number of the *ms* so implied are ever included in the awareness-unity relation. In all change of content, additions are accompanied by subtractions, so that while the number of factors making up the content may vary there is no marked expansion of content, and the infinite expansion implied in change and in the progress of knowledge is relative to awareness-unity bound up with a corresponding contraction. The limitation of content may be brought out then in various ways by reference to area, to change, to structure, etc., but to put it briefly it means that the conscious concretion or detail of content is in compass finite.

The ego–content theory has now been made over into the awareness-unity theory by emphasis on the primary and fundamental relations involved, and this has been done without recourse to the content theory or to behaviorism. The ego has been regarded as unimportant, and the content has been held to stand in what has been called the awareness-unity relation. To form an adequate conception of the awareness-unity theory the four factors of unity, awareness, content, and limitation must be taken together. Consciousness is first of all a unity of content, but unity and content even when taken together are not sufficiently specific. The unity of content might include the whole world. The unity must be the unity of a limited content, and this unity cannot be regarded as that part of the environment of the organism to which the organism is reacting, nor can it be regarded as the unity of the content of the present moment, because in either case the unity is determined through features of the content. The limitation of the unity of the content can only be determined and differentiated from that which lies beyond the unified content by the factor or relation called awareness. Now this relation, however vague and whatever it may be and whatever it may involve, can be verified as a fact and cannot be dispensed with. It is implied in feeling, knowing, and experiencing — though to say "I feel," or "I know," or "I experience," is misleading in attempting to define it, and to characterize it through such terms as immediacy, givenness, presence, light, apprehension, appearance, or even awareness, however suggestive those terms may be, is not to do justice to its real nature. All conceptions are suggested by content; therefore the conception of a relation which has nothing analogous to it or approximating it on the side of content is difficult to fathom. Unity and awareness supplement each other and they are again nothing without the limited content which they relate. Consciousness is then a unity of content limited by awareness, or it is a unifying awareness of limited content, or better still a limited awareness-unity of content.

In the foregoing criticism of the three fundamental theories as to the nature of mind a definite stand has been taken. On the one hand, behaviorism has been regarded as an inadequate and insufficient theory of mind, as a theory which leaves out of account much that may be properly called mental and which may even be regarded as the core of mind. As a study of the behavior of organisms it has been treated as a branch of biology rather than as psychology. On the other hand, mind has been thought of as essentially bound up with consciousness, and consciousness has been interpreted not according to the content theory as mere content, but in the light of the ego–content theory as including unity, awareness, content, and limitation. The ego has not been emphasized or even regarded as essential, yet those features which differentiate the content of consciousness from relations not included in the content have been retained. Mind being consciousness, and consciousness being a limited awareness-unity of content, how shall mind so conceived be determined? How is it to become the object of a science of psychology?

In connection with the conception of mind as a limited awareness-unity of content there are two facts to be borne in mind. In the first place, although unity is formal and awareness is colorless, and although the two taken together seem to be indifferent toward their content, awareness-unity has the advantage of being able to include anything within its content, any relation or system of relations, provided such relation or relations do not exceed the limitation of consciousness. Then, secondly, all color, all specific character, all relations except the relation which determines the limitation of content, all that gives any degree of concreteness to consciousness, belongs to content and is bound up with and determined by further relations or systems of relations beyond the content. Now it might seem, because the relations in the content are not determined by awareness-unity but are determined by the systems of relations in which they stand, that the relation of the relations in the content to consciousness is unimportant and superfluous, and that therefore there is no problem for psychology. But while the relations in the content are determined by the larger systems in which they stand, the fact that those relations fall within the content is not determined by such systems. In fact, the way in which relations fall under the awareness-unity relation, the way in which relations come within the limitation of content, suggests a problem not covered by the sciences concerned with the larger systems of relations. As this problem involves mind it is a problem for psychology and it may well be called *the* psychological problem. Psychology may then be said to be concerned with the problem of determining relations under the limitation of consciousness, and mind may be regarded as the object of psychology in so far as its content is studied as subject to its limitation. Stated in a more general way, psychology is the science of the relation of the object of truth to the mind.

The psychological problem is thus not to determine the nature of the mind by itself irrespective of anything else, but rather to determine the object of truth, including all possible relations as relative to the mind and its limitations. The *x* of psychology is not mere awareness-unity-content, it is any relation or relations as content of awareness-unity. Although the full working out of this conception of psychology must be left to the following chapters, four considerations should be here mentioned:

1. Any relations or objects may be content of consciousness. Awareness-unity only limits the number of factors in its content, not the quality or character of the content. Relations remote from each other in time and in space, universals and particulars, simple and complex objects, clearly outlined purposes and vague feelings, all may be included.

2. All relations or objects of truth are determined primarily through the systems of relations to which they belong. All content of consciousness therefore is determined irrespective of its status as content.

3. The relation of the objects of truth to consciousness is a further relation over and above the systems of relations in which the objects stand, and it is a relation secondary to those systems. Consequently the determination of this relation must come after the determination of the objects in their larger systems. The reconstructive method of description, and of course with it the non-causal method of explanation, is here suggested as the appropriate method for psychology.

4. In the reconstruction of the objects of truth as limited in consciousness, that is, in the determination of the content of consciousness, the various kinds of limitation must be defined and the different lines of research laid down.

CHAPTER IV

MIND AND TRUTH

THE PROBLEM OF THIS WORK is the problem of the problem of psychology. This may be expressed more directly by asking the question, what is psychology? To ask what is psychology is to ask what is mind, that is, what is the content or object of psychology. And to ask what is mind, is at least to ask what is truth, because the content or object of psychology can only be determined in the light of fundamental principles and relatively to other content of knowledge, and therefore relatively to the whole range and basis of knowledge, that is, to truth. Accordingly, in this work the conception of truth was first considered and found to be a progressive system of relations involving a foundation and including various sub-systems of relations which form the content of the various sciences. Then the conception of mind was studied, and after various views as to its nature were reviewed the theory that the mind is an awareness-unity of limited content was developed and accepted as valid. But to ask what psychology is, or more properly what psychology ought to be, is also to ask how psychology is related to the other branches of knowledge. This means to ask how its content or object, mind, is related to or finds its place in the whole content of truth. The place of psychology among the sciences can only be fixed by the determination of the status of mind in the system of truth. The next matter to be considered must then be the relation of mind to truth, the nature of mind in the light of truth and the various systems of truth. Only after the relation between mind and truth has been made clear can the proper content and method of psychology be defined.

In the study of the relation of mind to truth it should at the beginning be pointed out that the relation is a double one, for not only is mind to be understood in the light of truth but truth may be understood in the light of mind. Mind is an object or subject or content of truth having its place in the system of relations making up truth, and yet mind can know this system of relations. To make clear the place of mind in the system of relations, other objects of truth besides mind, and the relation of mind to those other objects as well as to the whole system of truth, must be defined and outlined. On this basis the relation of psychology to the other sciences and its place in the system of knowledge can be determined. But to relate mind to the other objects of truth implies consideration of the character of mind itself and above all of the unique character of mind that it can know truth. In fact, this character of mind in relation to truth must be defined before the place of mind among the other objects of truth can be fixed, its place in truth being in part dependent upon its nature.

The relation of mind to truth will be considered, then, first with respect to mind as knowing truth and afterwards with respect to the place of mind in truth and in relation to the other objects of truth.

For truth or any system of truth, mind is something additional. Whether truth is considered as structure or as a progressive system involving stages of knowledge, mind is always secondary and dependent but not presupposed by the structure or stages. Mind seems to be incidental to truth and comes to it as a sort of intuition of it, as being immediately conscious of it. In the account of the intuitional theory of truth it was pointed out that the intuition of the structure of truth added nothing to the structure although such intuition was important if mind were to know truth. In all research, in the study of truth's structure, in the push forward from positive knowledge into the *x* of knowledge, the intuition of structure and the plunge into the progressing knowledge are not factors which determine the result of such research. Yet they are added to truth, and the truth to which they are added forms the starting point for further progress in truth.

Truth, then, as structure, as a system of relations, and in its second dimension as stages of knowledge, is not fundamentally dependent on nor affected by intuition or consciousness, but mind as intuition of structure, as plunge into the progressive stages, as awareness-unity of truth, is in direct relation to truth without determining it. This relation is an important one for the conception of mind, and to understand it what might be called the freedom of truth must be made clear. In the development of the theory of truth in Chapter II three factors were distinguished: structure, knowledge, and knowing or mind. If truth rather than knowledge is the first consideration, then structure stands out as fundamental. In all its relations it seems to be that which truly is, — that which is valid beyond all question and which must be regarded as the ground or basis of the answer to all problems. But as structure is never complete and does not bring out the dynamic side of truth knowledge is added as a new dimension which represents the movement in the development of the structure. Knowledge means merely "truth on the march." It does not imply knowing or mind except as knowing is a further relation which does not affect structure and its development. Structure and knowledge must then be taken entirely objectively. If, on the other hand, knowledge is considered as the primary conception, then it is usually thought to have two sides or to point in two directions. It is thought to be a process or movement which involves both truth as structure and the mind which knows. It is, then, very easy to think that structure and mind involve each other, both being essential to knowledge. It is the fault of many idealists to regard the structure of truth as dependent on mind; or as they say, "object implies subject." No doubt knowledge is related to structure and to mind, but this does not mean that the relation between the structure and mind is such that the structure presupposes mind. It would be better to say, mind besides structure. The same would hold of the relation between knowledge and mind as knowing. Knowledge does not presuppose knowing, knowing being something beyond knowledge and not determining it. The idealist may be right as to the relation between knowledge and truth, but not as to the relation between knowledge and knowing.

Knowing is, then, a direct intuition of truth and knowledge, but it allows them their freedom. In other words, mind is (a) in direct relation to truth and knowledge (b) without influencing them, but is (c) suggestive of a further problem in addition to them. This problem may be more definitely suggested by pointing out that the truth or knowledge which is known or intuited may be a stage in the development of truth. Positive or actual knowledge known involves a knower or mind. But before the relation of the mind to the stages of knowledge can be studied the more general relation of truth and knowledge to mind as content of mind must be worked out.

For mind truth is content and content is an essential feature of mind. Though for truth mind may be an addendum, mind on its part includes truth and knowledge as part of its very structure, and would have no being without them. The four fundamental features of mind are unity, awareness, content, and limitation, but as content stands in relation to the other three features so does the truth which makes up the content. If mind is a limited awareness-unity of content or an awareness-unity of limited content it might also be said to be an awareness-unity of limited truth. How then is this limited truth related to awareness-unity? As for unity taken alone, it is very indefinite. It might be a mere group unity of the content, of the various relations which make up the truth, and unless further differentiated it might well include all truth. If mind were made up only of unity and content and therefore were nothing more than the unity of truth it would be a superfluous conception, because truth in its own nature as a system of relations includes such unity. With the addition of awareness to unity the situation is different. Awareness, though a feature of mind difficult to fathom, can be recognized as a feature or the feature which marks off content from non-content of consciousness. It was shown in Chapter III how there could be awareness of the fact that there were relations not included in the content of awareness. Awareness is therefore the basis for differentiating known truth from unknown truth and is the ground of the limitation of known truth as content of consciousness. Awareness as the ground of the limitation does not in itself define the details of known truth or the ways in which such truth is limited, but it does, together with unity, open up the psychological problem, the problem of mind in its connection with truth and knowledge.

Mind thus depends on truth but includes only part of it. Limited truth makes up the content of mind, and that such truth is limited is defined by awareness-unity. Furthermore, not only does awareness differentiate the known from the unknown, the content from the non-content of mind, but it expresses the direct or immediate relation of consciousness to the known truth. And this implies also that, just as unknown truth or non-content of mind is no part of mind, so there is no direct relation between mind and such truth or non-content. So far, then, as mind knows truth, two important relations stand out, the immediacy and the limitation of truth for mind. The result of the foregoing account of mind's relation to truth may be summed up in the statement that, while truth is not dependent on mind and mind is dependent on truth, mind includes only a limited part of truth but a part to which it stands in direct relation, the limitation of the truth and the directness of mind's relation to it being defined by awareness-unity. It is not as if truth were something given and by itself and mind also something given and by itself and that the two were then brought in relation to each other so that mind might be dependent on truth and yet in some way define its relation to truth. Mind is not external to truth, because truth is part of the structure of mind and mind adds something to truth. If mind is consciousness, it is the direct and limited consciousness of truth or a direct awareness-unity of limited truth.

A beginning of the conception of mind in relation to truth has now been outlined, and the basis for a fuller conception has been laid. But it may still be thought that the unity of consciousness is an indefinite and superfluous conception, that awareness is the differentiating conception, and that awareness of limited content is sufficient for the definition of consciousness. It may even be thought that awareness, too, though it is the differentiating feature between content and non-content, is superfluous and unimportant in that it adds nothing to the character of truth, and that therefore mind is primarily content and made up of truth and knowledge. It has been explained above that awareness must be added to unity, but it should here be pointed out that unity and awareness must be taken together. Not only is unity insufficient without awareness but awareness is insufficient without unity. Awareness alone may divide truth into content and non-content of consciousness, but so far as the content goes it can offer no further differentiating marks without unity. The whole content of which there is awareness makes up the field of positive knowledge, and all differences within it are matters defined by the content. If, however, unity and awareness are taken together it would not be possible to say that there is awareness-unity of all content, of all positive knowledge. There is awareness-unity of such content, but it is scattered in separate centers and not united in one awareness-unity. The whole difficulty with regard to the interrelations of the various features of mind may be cleared up by consideration of the various unities or degrees of unity involved.

First of all, there is the unity of all truth, including the whole system of possible and implied relations with all its subsystems and stages. This unity is centered and grounded in the logical core and covers all relations whether included in the *abc* or *x* of knowledge or in the content or non-content of mind. It is the all-inclusive unity of truth. Secondly, there is the unity of all positive knowledge or positive truth. It includes all that is known or determined and all that falls within the content as distinct from non-content of mind, it includes the *abc* and the *x* so far as the *x* is merely outlined and not determined in detail. It, too, is centered in the logical core but embraces what in Chapter II was called the epistemological core. As inclusive of all content it leaves out nothing which is known to mind, and as exclusive of all non-content it takes in all that falls under awareness. Then, thirdly, there is the unity of consciousness or unity of mind. It is a unity of content, awareness-unity. As a single feature of mind it is an empty conception, but as the unity or grouping of content which through awareness is distinguished from non-content it is most significant. This unity is not identical with the unity of positive knowledge. Undoubtedly all parts or phases of positive knowledge fall within the unity of consciousness, but no one unity of consciousness includes all positive knowledge. There may be a conscious unity of the general order of the unity of knowledge, and there may be conscious unities of various parts or details of knowledge. Such conscious unities, however, fall far short of the unity of positive knowledge and must be carefully distinguished from it. With the unity of consciousness carefully distinguished from the unity of positive knowledge and the unity of truth it is now possible to go on to show how the unity of consciousness when taken in connection with content and awareness is crucial in defining mind.

The unity of truth has little to offer by way of determining the conception of mind; it merely points to the totality of truth. Positive knowledge as distinct from its unity falls within the content of mind, but to be content rather than non-content is unimportant. The marking off of the content of truth from non-content on the basis of awareness is at most the dividing of truth into two parts. Not only does awareness add nothing to truth in making it content, awareness being neutral and not affecting truth, but the division of truth into content and non-content has no value for positive knowledge, since the non-content is the unknown, the *x*, the not-yet-determined. Furthermore, the full unity of positive knowledge lies beyond knowledge and content, because there is no knowledge of all details known and of all content brought together in one unity. However contradictory it may seem, it is quite correct to say that positive knowledge is not known. Every detail may be known, and its unity may be known in general outline, but the complete unity including all detail is not known. The conception of mind cannot be defined, then, in any satisfactory way by means of the conceptions of truth, or content, or awareness, or by means of any or of all of these taken together, nor can it be defined by the conception of unity when taken alone. Unity, awareness, and content must be taken together. Awareness may differentiate content from non-content and so mark off the field for mind, but without unity there would be no consciousness and therefore no mind or minds. One of the great mistakes in the understanding of mind as consciousness lies in finding its differentiating mark either in unity or in awareness but not in both. Limited awareness-unity of content is the minimum of mind.

The limitation of awareness-unity of content means the limitation of truth which is content or knowledge on the basis of awareness, and the further limitation of knowledge on the basis of unity. This awareness-unity of content defines mind, or rather, minds. The content might be referred to as the immediate object of consciousness. It is that which is given, not the given as contrasted with constructions of the mind but as the full content, including acts of volition, images, and feelings as well as conceptions, perceptions, sensations, etc. Truth, then, as content, as given, as immediate object of consciousness, is an integral part of mind. It might even be said that mind is truth subjected to the limitations of awareness-unity. Truth is free and determinable independently, but the grouping of truth in consciousness is a matter for further determination, and this grouping is central to mind.

Much has been said to ward off misconceptions of the nature of mind and of its fundamental features in their relations to one another. With these features and their interrelations clarified, it ought now to be possible to gain further insight into the conception of mind in relation to truth. Mind may be defined as an awareness-unity of limited content, or as the immediately given truth of awareness-unity, or again as the grouping and massing of truth and knowledge in consciousness. Truth is related to mind as its limited immediate object, and the study of mind is the study of this object in its immediacy and under its limitation. These two features of immediacy and limitation must be borne in mind; they must be taken together and can only be considered together.

Though the limited immediate object might be any phase of truth, because of its limitation it may be very warped and insignificant as an expression of truth. As the limitation is a limitation to a relatively small number of factors in the content, the factors might be such as to suggest a wide range with few details of the object of truth or they might be a group of details of some particular object or part of truth and exclusive of its more general pattern. In either case the truth as truth may be distorted, and there are some strata of truth which can never be included in any adequate way in the content of consciousness. Beside possible objects which lie beyond consciousness and have no connection with the content of consciousness, it may be said that the object of consciousness as built out and completed in all its relations is never content of consciousness. There is no awareness-unity of an unlimited object. It may furthermore be said that there is no consciousness of all the stages of truth and knowledge or of any final stage which might supplement and correct the earlier stages. The mind is always confined to a stage, although it may move on to a further stage. In fact the limited immediate object is not highly concrete.

The unreflecting mind may think that it sees or is conscious of objects in their full concreteness. But the detail of objects in perception is very limited. The man sitting at his desk senses very little of it in his perception. He is conscious of its general shape and texture, that it offers resistance to his hands, and he has a vague sense of its purpose, but these factors are a very small part of what the desk is as an object, and the perceptions which the man has of the desk during the day make up very little of the desk as an object lasting throughout the day. The present time in which the man lives is again a very small part of the complete time, including past, present, and future, and the remembered or imagined event is relatively meagre in its content. Also in the conception of a star, or of a law of nature, most of the particulars which fall under the conception are not included in consciousness. It may therefore be said that although mind's content as including connected and related elements is essentially synthetic and concrete, it never includes any highly complex object or intricate group of relations in full detail. This limited immediate object being immediate as well as limited, it may now be asked how far the immediacy of the object carries. In the partially concreted object of perception there could be no question as to its immediacy. The sensations in the perception are directly given or present to consciousness, and the order and arrangement of the elements in the object of perception are also given. It may be impossible to explain any particular order or arrangement without reference to past experience or to perceptions no longer present, but as to the perceived object itself it is clearly present. If the perceived object is thought to refer to some further object beyond perception, the reference cannot be made on the basis of perception alone; therefore any such further object is no true part of the perceived object, which is immediate. Space and time are both important features in the order of perception, but while the limited space included in the object of perception may vary very much, time is limited to the present. The present as exclusive of the past and the future is the duration of perception included within the so-called "time-span," and the very brief duration included in the time-span is relatively constant as compared with the variations in space-perception. However limited perception is, it is generally recognized as immediately given in consciousness. In fact it is regarded as essentially given or present, as the immediate *par excellence*. But it is a more difficult matter to bring out immediacy in connection with other phases of the mind.

In regard to memory of past events, most psychologists would say that an image is present in consciousness and represents or refers to some past event, this past event not being immediately given. The question naturally arises as to how the image refers to the past event. If it is said to be like that event, that is, to represent it or to correspond to it, difficulty as to the correspondence appears because the image cannot be compared with the past event if there is no awareness-unity of that event. If some method or plan of connecting the image with the past event is suggested, this plan or connection must include the event; and the plan including the event must in some way be given in consciousness. It is not necessary that all the details of the past event as originally experienced be regarded as given, only some feature or relation in the event is needed. The event and the image need not be separated; it is sufficient to regard the image as including some part of the original concretion, though it is not so fully concrete as the original. Along with some consciousness, however vague, that this concretion belongs in the past, there may be many features in the image which have no place in the past, and there generally are many sensations and feelings in the background of the content of consciousness which have no place in the concretion belonging to the past.

Consider, for example, the case of a man who remembers a flood which he experienced as a boy. He remembers being awakened in the night, rushing downstairs half dressed, being taken shivering and trembling in a boat to a place of safety, and then being crowded into a public building until morning. His fear which he experienced at the time of the flood and his sorrow at the possible loss of his toys play a very small part in his memory, though a pleasurable feeling in remembering the event, accompanied by a certain emotional excitement in telling of it, is present. Now his image of the past events fits more or less accurately into a place in his past life. The past is for him a conception or plan of a series of completed events stretching back from the present. Its detail is very meagre and it may be thought of as a line or a numerical series or as a continuum of happenings of which relatively few come to mind. The plan or conception and some detail of the remembered image make up the minimum of memory. A feeling of pastness may possibly also be included. It is however important to note that the various features of the memory image truly belong in the past, for instance, the peculiar squeak of the oars in the oarlocks, or the color of the clothes of some of the people sitting in the public building. These features have their proper place in past time, and the consciousness of them on the part of the man who remembers them is an immediate consciousness of something in past time. The features, color or sound, are not, then, repetitions of former sensations. In immediate consciousness they may fall within the same awareness-unity with certain features which may be regarded as belonging to present time, for instance, the pleasurable feeling accompanying the memory of the thrilling experience. The color or sound, therefore, stands in two contexts, both falling within one awareness-unity. The color or sound has its place in the past and in the present, but because it is connected with present features it should not be regarded as *referring only* to the past or as *merely representative* of the past. The upshot of this view of memory is to bring out the fact that there is immediate awareness-unity or consciousness of past events, though the content of these past events may include very small bits of the past.

The same holds with the imaginative forecast of the future as with memory, so far as the future can be foreseen, but so far as the future is not determinable any imaginative construction of it is merely a possibility and subject to correction like a hypothesis which may have to be discarded.

If memory, then, may be said to be a direct consciousness of the past, and if imagination taken in its most general sense may be said to include all content not present in sensation or in perception, conception may be regarded as including all or any content whatsoever, whether present or past, whether temporal in character or not. As not conditioned by time, it may be thought of as trans-temporal or super-temporal or non-temporal. The concept of a star or an atom includes something characteristic of all stars or atoms, past, present, and future. The concept of a law of nature includes a function which may take place at any or all times in nature, and the concept of justice is one which holds irrespective of time. The concept of time itself, while not strictly speaking in time or conditioned by time, contains or includes a minimum of the framework of time. Furthermore, a concept when thought of as a universal character or relation should not be regarded as an abstraction from concrete detail, but rather as a starting point or beginning of such concretion. The interesting fact which ought now to be obvious is that neither in memory, nor in imagination, nor in conception is the content of consciousness limited to the present; it expands far beyond present sensation, perception, and feeling. While the content of consciousness is limited in amount of detail, the detail is not confined to that of present time. The limited immediate content of awareness-unity might be then almost anything provided it does not reach too high a degree of concretion.

It is a mistake to think of the world as a manifold of absolute things or concrete events spread out through time and to think of consciousness as likewise an event in time centered largely in the time at which it takes place, just as it is a mistake to build up the conception of mind on the basis of sensation, perception, and feeling as present data and to regard the other functions of mind as emanating from these functions or as being extensions of them. That the empirical self[1] is defined through certain present sensations and feelings in the background of consciousness should not be misleading. That $7 + 5 = 12$ is always the same $7 + 5 = 12$, and that a detail of truth such as a color, or a group of details or relations, is the same detail or group irrespective of time, would probably be generally accepted; and in the same way the placing of such detail in its proper place in time, whether in past, present, or future, and the beginning in the content of consciousness of the plan for its setting, ought also to be recognized as equally valid and eternal. Consciousness, then, may be very confined and very sketchy but its span is not limited to the time-span of perception.

From the conception that the content of consciousness is given and immediate relative to awareness-unity rather than to present time, two important consequences follow. In the first place, consciousness is not in time, time is in consciousness. If consciousness were in time and limited in time, it would not be possible for time to be content of consciousness,

[1] James, *The Principles of Psychology*, I, 291–305; Marshall, *Consciousness*, pp. 3, 4, 36, 480–523.

though particular sequences in time might be such content. Memory of past time, imaginative forecast of future time, and in fact any conception of time as an order would be out of the question. Secondly, there is change in the content of consciousness which is not temporal change. For instance, suppose a mind brings to the focus of its content part of some experience of yesterday, then turns to part of some experience of a year ago, and then considers the conception of justice. So far as these contents go they do not follow in temporal sequence. The first comes after the second in time, and the third is not in time at all. If there were no further content, no content in the background, it could not be said that these contents named follow each other according to any time order. Though it may be said that the full content of consciousness reveals sensations and feelings flowing in temporal sequence and that the contents above mentioned being connected with them must be thought to partake of that sequence, there seems to be no good reason why the kind of sequence found in part of the content should define the sequence for some other part of the content of consciousness. Why should sensation and feeling be definitive? The view here maintained is that conscious change as a phase of the limitation of content is relative to awareness-unity and therefore may or may not be temporal change or change according to any temporal order.

In the light of what has here been advanced it may now be asked whether behaviorism and the content theory are satisfactory theories. Can past experience, or can time, be explained on the basis of either one of these two theories?

According to behaviorism, mind is centered in the functions of the brain. The brain being in space–time all its functions take place in space–time. Any detail of events which took place in past time or which are taking place outside of the brain, or any moral concept which might have no primary reference to space–time, might be represented in the functions of the brain. But it would have to be represented and not given immediately to the brain. One part of space–time could hardly include any other part of space–time or that which is not in space–time though it might easily contain features representative of that which is beyond itself. In fact any detail which might appear in the content of consciousness could in some way be represented in the functions of the brain. To accept behaviorism would be to go back to the representative or correspondence theory of truth, and then a question would arise as to how the representation is to be compared with the original. Of course it might still be said that the mind as the functioning of the brain could neglect those functions so far as they were in a particular place and time and could emphasize those functions which referred beyond. Still, the referring functions would be in a particular part of space–time. The functions of the brain are hardly adequate to any super-temporal conception of mind.

A similar difficulty is to be found with the content theory. According to this theory, mind is merely content and the content is in time. Now the content of some particular time can hardly be said to include content of other times or content which is not in time. Like the functions of the brain, it might represent content beyond itself and it might minimize the fact that it is in a particular time. But if such content is to know content of other times or non-temporal content it can only do so by representation. The difficulty of the representative theory again appears. And if some partisan of the content theory should maintain that the content can include non-temporal features or features of past time, then the content theory approaches the awareness-unity theory; but without awareness and unity it has no means of explaining the extent and limitation of content.

It ought now to be clear that the unity of the brain and of its functions and the unity of the present moment in time are not sufficient to express the unity of the mind. The content of the mind is more than temporal and includes transitions which are not primarily temporal. The unity of its content must thus be a very far-reaching one, although not full in detail. It ought also to be clear that awareness is neither a function of the brain nor a phase of content. It is unfortunate to say that awareness is "a relation of something to something else, such that the attributes of content result," having "no positive characteristics," and being "adequately accounted for by any physical process which will account for the attributes of content." [2] Awareness is undoubtedly an indefinable relation relative to content and is that which distinguishes content from non-content, but there is no reason for identifying it with content nor for regarding it as explainable by processes which may explain content. Awareness and unity belong together, and taken together they stand over against content, the content being free as to its structure and not by itself sufficient to define mind.

The mind in knowing truth only begins to know truth through its content. In any stage of knowledge a mind can be said only to have made a start at knowing truth, to have included within its content a very small part of knowledge. It is not correct to think of parcels of truth as being given from which the mind may be said to abstract certain general relations. It would be more correct to speak of the mental process of knowing as a kind of subtraction rather than abstraction, that is, as a subtracting of the irrelevant detail and of connecting those features which form what is essential to the object of knowledge. Whether in perception, imagination, or conception the mind interprets its content by building out and concreting its object, not by starting with a ready-made concretion.

Granted, then, that mind is not limited to any part of space–time or to present time, it should be pointed out that an important feature of mind appears in the conception of the individual center of consciousness or the individual awareness-unity of limited content. The conception of the individual was discussed as a conception used in defining mind and the psychical world, and it was found to be inadequate; but it now appears as a valuable conception in bringing out one of the limitations of mind. Consciousness is always an awareness-unity of a content which is a very small part of the field of positive knowledge. There are unities of all parts of positive knowledge and there is awareness of all parts, but there is no

[2] Karl Spencer Lashley, "The Behavioristic Interpretation of Consciousness," *Psychological Review* (Princeton), xxx (1923), 329.

one awareness-unity of all of it. Awareness-unity is split up into separate centers, and consciousness is always to be found in such centers, therefore the massing of truth as the content of awareness-unity involves massing in individual conscious centers.

Reference to the individual here is not intended to mean reference either to the organism or to the ego. Nor is it intended to refer solely to the content of consciousness. Although two individual centers of consciousness could not be distinguished except by their content, the individual consciousness is meant to include both unity and awareness as well as content.

In all that has now been said with regard to the relation of truth to mind, with regard to mind knowing truth, certain important relations stand out. Truth is related to mind directly and immediately but subject to very decided limitations. While on the one hand the range of objects of truth which may be immediately given to mind is very great, on the other hand the number of objects, the amount of concretion, which may be given is very small. What has been said with regard to the range and limitation of the immediate may be summed up as follows:

1. Truth and knowledge are given immediately and not by representation to awareness-unity as its content. They are systems of relations not in themselves involving consciousness yet necessary to its make-up.

2. Most varied parts of truth and knowledge, most diverse relations and groups of relations, may be given to awareness-unity. Its range covers objects of perception, memory, imagination, and conception, objects near and distant in space and time, objects of moral and aesthetic value; indeed any relation may be included within its purview.

3. The number of relations or factors of truth and knowledge given to awareness-unity is always limited. Whatever features of truth and knowledge fall within consciousness as given, they form a relatively small group, thus narrowing the concretion of truth before the mind to very confined areas. This statement is little more than the limitation of the con-

tent of awareness-unity in terms of truth rather than in terms of content.

4. The given relations of truth and knowledge are limited to individual centers of consciousness. Not only are the number of relations limited, but such limited groups of relations are in separate individual consciousnesses, forming many distinct individual groupings.

5. Though the grouping and massing of truth and knowledge in consciousness and in separate centers of consciousness is limited, the change of content relative to awareness-unity, that is, its non-temporal change, makes possible an extension, a development, and a selection of the factors grouped in the mind such as could not be attained in a single grouping of relations of truth. The more fundamental relations of truth in their important connections can in this way be brought to consciousness, the breadth of view of the mind not being checked by its limitation.

It may now be said that mind is truth within the limits of awareness-unity, and that such truth may be very diverse and involve wide perspective. In place, then, of the definition of mind as an awareness-unity of limited content, the definition of it may be given as an awareness-unity of limited truth or knowledge. But at once objection will be made that truth, or even knowledge, is not an appropriate characterization of all content of consciousness. It will be claimed that many phases of the content are not included under truth; that feeling, emotion, volition, and other parts of the content of the mind are not truth or knowledge. In fact it may be thought that this whole approach to mind on the basis of truth and knowledge is misleading, and that knowledge and truth are not fundamental but incidental to mind, and incidental only to minds of a relatively high order. In answer to this objection it may be said, though truth and knowledge are not commonly used to characterize all the content of mind, that the content is made up of relations, and as truth is a system of relations and comprehensive of all relations it is not inappropriate to refer to the content of mind as truth or as part of truth or possibly as an object of truth.

It is also not inappropriate to refer to the content as knowledge, in as much as the content as composed of relations falls within the general field of positive knowledge, though all its details may not as yet have been determined. The mind which is conscious of feeling, emotion, or volition may not have knowledge of them in the full sense, it may not be aware of them as phases of truth or of some system of truth, it may not express them in judgmental or propositional form, but this does not mean that they do not stand in relation to some system of truth or knowledge. Furthermore, as they stand in such relation to truth, it is not possible to give any full account of mind without taking account of those relations, and therefore of truth and knowledge in their larger aspects. Mind may here be approached from the intellectual side, but no determination of the content of mind can be made in any other way. The broader conception of truth and knowledge is logically prior to the narrow and more limited conception of any part of it, and the content of mind cannot be understood apart from the systems of truth to which it belongs.

It might further be objected that awareness-unity as brought out in Chapter III is vague and of little value in the determination of the mind, and that it is the will that gives to the mind its unity through the determination of truth as the mind's content. For instance, Royce regards the will as of primary significance in any conception of truth. He says, "no idea is true or is false except with reference to the object that this very idea first means to select as its own object." [3] In other words, the intention or the will is fundamental. The answer to this objection ought to be clear. Though the will may select or intend or mean certain parts of truth, though in the determination of truth the mind may always consciously aim at some object to be known, it is not the will but the structure of the truth which makes the truth what it is. In the activity of the mind in consciously striving to obtain truth the will may be an important feature, but it is not essential to the truth which it seeks, nor is it a factor in the nature of truth at which it aims. However valuable the

[3] Josiah Royce, *The World and The Individual* (New York, 1900–01), I, 31.

will may be in the search for truth and in the moral life, it is not the only function or content of the mind, and therefore, if other phases of truth beside the will belong to the content of the mind, it cannot be the fundamental unity of the mind. Awareness-unity may be a vague conception, particularly because awareness is difficult to define, but it is certainly a more inclusive unity of the mind than any unity of the will. There are, it then appears, two dangers: first, that the will be regarded as the basis of truth and knowledge, and second, that the will rather than awareness-unity be thought to give mind its primary unity. But as has been shown, the will is neither the structural unity of truth nor *the* unity of the mind.

Early in this chapter it was pointed out that mind as an object of truth has its place in the systems of relations making up truth, and that at the same time it may know those relations, and its knowing those relations must be considered in determining its place among them and therefore in defining its relation to truth. It was then necessary to bring out the relation of truth to mind as mind's content, mind knowing truth, before taking up the place of mind in the system of truth. As the relation of mind knowing truth has now been considered, the study of the place of mind in the system of truth may be undertaken.

If the relation of truth to mind could be thought of as the relation of a box to its cover or as a river to its banks it would be a relatively simple matter to understand the relation, but a spatial analogy can hardly be used to bring out the relation of truth to mind. The relation is a peculiarly intimate one. The box is not the cover and the river is not the river bank, but truth is an integral part of mind and its relations make up mind's content. Yet in spite of this intimacy of truth and mind, truth is not merely the content or merely one of the ingredients of mind. If it were, it would not be difficult to understand this relation. But truth has a structure of its own and is made up of a very elaborate system of relations, and in so far as it is not the truth of mind its structure is not determined by mind. Therefore, in the determination of the place of mind in truth the general structure of truth is primary and the relations which make up mind are secondary. In other words, it should be remembered on the one hand that the content of mind is truth; that truth, though in limited amount, stands in direct relation to mind; and that most diverse systems and regions of truth may be so related; while on the other hand the body and structure of truth as well as its major systems are largely independent, and as it depends on them for its content it must be studied after they have been outlined or determined. However closely, then, psychology is related to the other branches of truth, it is a secondary or subordinate science.

To make clear the way in which the immediate relation of mind to truth and the dependence of mind on truth go together, it should be pointed out that the content of mind is first truth and then content. That it is content does not make it what it is but merely signifies that it falls within awareness-unity. The awareness-unity of limited truth is an addition to the truth taken by itself. A mind conscious of a star or an atom or of a moral principle or a beautiful landscape is something more than those objects of truth, and yet without them or other objects of which it might be conscious it would be nothing. Mind thus presupposes some object or objects or some truth. But if it be asked what more mind is than these objects it is only possible to turn to the conceptions of unity, awareness, and the limitation of truth as content.

Some truth being presupposed as the condition of mind and as its immediate content, the concept of unity by itself has little to offer, because it might be said to be contained in the truth or object; but awareness, or better, awareness combined with unity, may suggest an addition. Awareness or awareness-unity of a truth or object is more than the truth or object by itelf. Yet it may be questioned whether this more is of any real consequence. Suppose it be admitted that mind may be defined through unity, awareness, and content, it may at the same time be held that awareness, like unity, is always the same, and that therefore it is only the content which needs to be considered; and as the content is an object of truth, it should properly be determined as a phase of truth and not as a phase of mind. Mind might then seem to be neutral and unimportant and perhaps not a significant object of truth.

Possibly something may be made of mind on the basis of the conception of knowledge. Positive knowledge can be defined as the knowledge which falls within the content as distinct from the non-content of mind. This content is defined by awareness. Therefore, awareness might be thought to be important in determining positive knowledge. Philosophy, science, or knowledge is content of mind. No matter how far content contains implications of non-content or suggestions as to any plan regarding its nature, all such implications and suggestions belong to content. Yet as non-content lies beyond knowledge the distinction between content and non-content on the basis of awareness might well be said to make no difference to knowledge. The most that awareness can do would then seem to be to mark off knowledge but not to make any distinctions within the field of knowledge.

There is, of course, beside the conception of positive knowledge, the conception of progressive knowledge, of "truth on the march." It might at first sight seem as if the progress of knowledge were mental while the truth was to be found in the content and that therefore the movement of knowledge might be the mental factor to be added to the given truth. But it should not be forgotten that truth is also progressive and that any knowledge of it to which the mind progresses is also content. Even the earlier stages of knowledge which might be reconstructed are both truth and content. Yet the distinction between the movement of the mind in knowledge and the movement of truth is a genuine one and is suggestive of one phase of the problem of mind. If it be asked how the mind progresses, that is, how it organizes and masses its progressing knowledge, the problem as to the conditions and limitations of consciousness is involved. This consideration leads back to the more general conception of the limitation of the content of consciousness, but it does suggest that the limitation of content should be taken to include the limitations of a moving and changing consciousness.

In view of the foregoing considerations, namely, that mind is secondary to truth as a kind of additional truth, that the distinction between content and non-content is unimportant and unity and awareness add little that is significant, and that the movement of consciousness is not the distinguishing mark of mind, it may be said that positive truth or knowledge as content of awareness-unity by being such content acquires no significant additional truth except for the way in which it is massed and limited under awareness-unity. Not the mere falling of truth and knowledge within consciousness, but the conditions and limitations of truth in consciousness, make up the mental factor of truth, the additional mental truth which gives mind its place in truth. This grouping and massing of the limited content of mind forms the subject matter of psychology.

In the characterization of consciousness in Chapter III as involving the four features of unity, awareness, content, and the limitation of content it was stated that the limitation of content meant that the factors making up the detail of the content of awareness-unity were limited in number. This is an expression of the limitation of content in its most general form, but this limitation appears in various ways so that various kinds of limitation must be distinguished.

In the first place there is the limitation of the span of consciousness. By this is meant that the number of factors in the content included under one awareness-unity is finite. This limitation emphasizes the single awareness-unity of content in its full extent and concretion. It may be differentiated into two different kinds, as the span of consciousness seems to have two phases. There is the span of perception and the span of imagination. The span of perception is limited in time to the present in what is generally spoken of as the time-span. The content falling within the time-span is limited both with respect to its extension in space and with respect to the number of elements included within it. These elements are composed chiefly of sensations, relations among sensations

— including spatial and temporal relations, and feelings. The span of imagination, though also limited as to the number of elements within its span, is not confined within the time-span but includes very varied non-perceptual content, such as remembered and constructed objects, universal and particular concepts, ideas, intentions, etc. In the former case it is given and present, while in the latter it is given but not necessarily present, but in both cases it is given in one single span of awareness-unity.

Secondly, there is the limitation connected with change in consciousness. The content of consciousness is always undergoing alteration. New factors constantly appear in consciousness and then disappear from it. Though there may be a gain in moving from one stage of consciousness to another and so breaking the bounds of a single awareness-unity of content, the loss of many factors of the content of the earlier stage from the later stage imposes a real limitation. Problems may be solved and more factors may be added but no great accretions or accumulations of detail can be retained as content. This kind of limitation is merely an extension of the first kind mentioned so that account may be taken of change in consciousness. It might be said that the span of perception involves a limitation in the loss of present factors which pass into the past, and that the span of imagination is limited in a similar way. And it should be added that the mind cannot sweep on *ad libitum* from one stage to all future stages, but must move forward stage by stage, thus the not-yet, the future, as well as the past, imposes its barrier. The content of awareness-unity, while always changing, is, then, prevented from expansion by the gradual character of its changing process and by its actual loss of content.

Thirdly, there is the limitation not in the number of factors in consciousness but in the division of the factors themselves. In any attempt to break up or analyze the factors of the content of consciousness into their simpler parts or elements, elements are found which cannot be divided or broken up any further, for example: in perception the quality of a pure color or the *minimum visibile* of a colored field, or the intensity of pleasure in feeling. In imagination, although the division of the factors, like their composition, is freer and therefore more easily penetrated by analysis, elements do appear which cannot be further divided, as in the case of an image of a pure color or sound, in the concept of unity, or in the relation of difference. Some of these unanalyzed elements may be composite, but mind cannot penetrate them directly as they stand given in the content of consciousness. This limitation in the division of factors must not be overlooked, for it is fully as important as that of the span of consciousness, or of the limitation connected with change.

The first and second kinds of limitation may well be spoken of as the higher or upper limit, while the third kind may be spoken of as the lower limit of the content. Between these two limits the consciousness is decidedly hemmed in.

Fourthly, there is a kind of limitation due to the number of individual consciousnesses which include in their content the same object of truth. In the consciousness of any truth or object on the part of more than one individual consciousness, the detail of the object or truth is not the same in the various consciousnesses of which it is content, and it is not massed in the same way in these various consciousnesses. The unity, for instance, of one whole system of truth with all its detail, the whole of positive knowledge in any one field, is never all included under one awareness-unity. Such detail and points of view of the system as are given in the various individual centers of consciousness can be so diverse that they might almost seem not to be parts of one system. This limitation has particular significance in the higher ranges of knowledge.

As a corollary to what has just been said it should be pointed out in the phenomena of attention and will where a high degree of discrimination and concentration is involved that with the selection of certain factors other factors are driven out of the content of consciousness. In this way limitation is brought about through the complication of features within the content.

At this point the secondary character of psychological truth should again be pointed out. If a limitation is to be defined, or if limits are to be marked off, the appropriate procedure is to lay out the whole field first and then to impose the limitations. Accordingly, the logical course in determining truth would be to study the larger systems of truth first and then to determine how these systems are limited as content of awareness-unity, as relative to mind. Logic, physical science, moral science, aesthetics, and other objective branches of truth stand first in line. Psychology as the science of mind then follows, accepting the content of these sciences and determining how that content is the content of mind. Its method is essentially reconstructive. Mental truth is an addition to all other truths by bringing that truth within the confines of awareness-unity and thereby adding to all other truth the truth of such other truth's limitation in consciousness. The whole field of knowledge includes the objective systems of truth plus their relation to mind.

In Chapter II knowledge was referred to as a kind of second dimension of truth, as suggesting its dynamic aspect. Knowledge at any one stage tends to move on to further stages. Now this forward movement of knowledge is always a forward movement of positive knowledge, knowledge falling under awareness. The movement of knowledge to obtain more and more truth is a movement of further and further penetration into the object of truth. It might be spoken of as the objective tendency in knowledge. Natorp has called this tendency the objective direction of knowledge, and he has called the movement in the opposite direction back to earlier stages the subjective direction. According to his view, if the latest stage attained in positive knowledge be taken as a starting point, that stage with its tendency to press forward to further stages would be regarded as falling within the field of objective science or constructive knowledge, while the attempt to reconstruct or go back to prior stages of knowledge would fall within the subjective field, the field of psychology.[4] This moving back to earlier stages would not be a matter of genetics nor of history but rather a reëstablishment of the general out-

[4] Natorp. *Allgemeine Psychologie nach kritischer Methode*, pp. 189–213, 229–262.

lines of those stages. Now the recognition of the objective movement in knowledge is important, and the suggestion that the reconstruction of earlier stages of knowledge is a psychological problem cannot be overemphasized. It does not seem however that this problem is the central psychological problem nor definitive of psychological science, for not only are the earlier stages objective as well as subjective or mental, but the latest stage is subjective as well as objective, since it is knowledge and therefore content of mind. The dynamic aspect of truth as knowledge can, then, hardly be used to define the mental or psychical.

The relation of mind or psychological truth to other truth has now been outlined in its fundamental character. It may be summed up as follows: Truth is a synthetic structure, a system of relations including a central core of primary and fundamental relations and also a vast detail of relations which fall into various sub-systems. This structure is dynamic; it is a changing and developing system and moving forward from stage to stage, such forward movement being due to the necessity and implications of the structure. On the one hand, no absolute or ultimate truth, no completed structure, can be attained; truth is essentially flowing. The only determinable truth is the truth of a stage. The aim of knowledge is to press forward from stage to stage with a view to defining the object of truth as fully as possible. This objective and dynamic tendency of knowledge is characteristic of it and may be spoken of as the second dimension of truth. The various types of object toward which knowledge is directed may be classed as logical, imaginary, physical, psychological, ontological, technical, moral, and aesthetic. These types of object define the various problems and sub-systems of knowledge, and with the exception of the psychological object express the general lines of objectification in knowledge. On the other hand, this dynamic system of truth is not just mental, not merely a knowing on the part of the mind, not merely content of consciousness. Truth as structure, as a system of relations, is more than mental content; and as a changing structure it cannot be identified with the change of content in mind. Objective truth is therefore neither ultimate nor mental. In contrast, however, with all purely objective forms of truth, mind stands out as the object or subject of psychological truth. Any objective truth or body of truth may be the content or immediate object of mind, and the conditions under which it falls within the bounds of mind and forms its content make up the detail of psychological truth. This psychological truth is, of course, objective in the sense that it is valid, but unlike the primary or pure objective truth it depends on that other truth and is secondary to it. As secondary and dependent, its relation to other truth must be taken account of, and particularly its relation to the various branches and sub-systems of knowledge. From the point of view of mind, truth is its food; from the point of view of truth, mind is a dependent thing; and for knowledge, psychology is the last science. If the method of objective science is the interpretation or explanation of the various objects or branches of truth, the method of psychological science is the further interpretation or explanation of those objects as relative to mind, as in immediate relation to consciousness. Thus if objective science may be spoken of as constructive, psychology is reconstructive.

The relation of psychological truth to objective truth in general having now been outlined, its relation to the various systems or sub-systems of truth remains to be considered. Some account must be given of the relation of psychology to logic, of the relation of mind to the primary principles of truth, and of the sub-systems of truth. Strictly speaking, logic is not the science of a sub-system but rather of the super-system or skeleton of all systems. But as such a science is concerned with principles and relations of great importance, its relation to psychology can hardly be neglected. As for the imaginary systems, the value of which lies in bringing out the range of possible systems which may be based on the logical superstructure, to them no special attention need be given since their relation to mind adds little which does not appear in connection with the relation of mind to other sub-systems. Mathematical systems based on freely chosen postulates, ideal moral systems, realities unrelated to the known world, and self-contradictory systems, though freer and less tied down to details than real or teleological systems, have little to suggest relative to mind and its determination which is not included in these other systems. Real systems in contrast with imaginary systems have an important bearing on mind. Psychology cannot be considered apart from these systems, in fact, it is the science of one such system or sub-system. Real systems have to do with realities, existences, actualities, with details or phenomena not included in or fully defined by the logical core, and in general they exclude that which is merely possible as well as the normative or teleological systems. Real systems or sub-systems seem to be of three sorts as based on the physical problem of the space–time world, the psychological problem of mind, and the ontological problem of the ultimate framework of reality as a whole. Because of the close relation of these three spheres to each other, an account of the relation of psychology both to physical science and to ontology cannot be left unconsidered. The relation of mind to the teleological or ideal systems is also important. If the teleological systems be divided into technical, moral, and aesthetic, it should be noted that technical problems involve a large amount of detail and that the aesthetic problem is complicated and at the present time highly controversial. Therefore technical and aesthetic systems will be left out of account, but the moral world or system will be considered and taken as typical of teleological systems. The relation of psychology to ethics or moral philosophy will then be included in the following account. The relation of psychology to logic, to physical science, to ethics, and to ontology will be taken up, and in the order here named.

To make clear the relation of psychology to logic means to study the relation of mind to the logical core. The logical core is made up of the fundamental conditions or relations of all truth together with the fundamental relations of the sub-systems of truth. Such relations as those of unity, difference, implication, order, causality, existence, law, etc., would be included among the fundamental relations. These fundamental relations belong essentially to the structure of truth and make up its formal framework. They are not to be regarded as mental products or principles although mind may be conscious of them. As independent of mind they still do not stand by themselves but hang together with the whole system of truth as its necessary condition or *sine qua non*. The detail of truth presupposes the framework, both framework and detail being interrelated in the structure. The fundamental relations of the core might be spoken of as the postulates of truth, and as in the march of truth from stage to stage truth's structure may change, the postulates may change in harmony with the changing structure. These postulates or fundamental relations, which form primarily the framework of truth, are at the same time directly related to mind. Mind may be immediately conscious of the fundamental relations as conditioning and as belonging to the system or systems of truth. This immediate consciousness of fundamentals implies that the representative theory with regard to the relation of logical principles to the mind must be ruled out. But if mind can grasp the framework of an independent truth, how can it bring that framework within the limited content of consciousness? Neither the framework as a whole nor the framework in its relation to the structure of truth can be brought within a single content of awareness-unity. There may be no difficulty in relating a single fundamental relation to consciousness, but consciousness of this fundamental relation with all that it conditions seems impossible. The question then arises as to the conditions under which a limited mind may know logical principles. A study of these conditions is a kind of psychology of logic, or a psychology of the logical as distinct from logic itself.

It is common to regard concept, judgment, inference, and reasoning as the primary forms in which truth is expressed in the mind, as the highest mental forms in which it is given in consciousness, and consequently as the forms in which logical principles are expressed. To these may be added volition and perception, also possibly sensation, desire, and feeling. Volition does not in its primary function express truth, but so far as it does so it would fall under concept or judgment or possibly under perception. Perception, while distinct from conception, does seem to express truth and to involve a measure of judgment; but it is distinctly concrete in character and expresses no universal principles. Therefore the fundamental relations of the logical core, while implied, are not expressed in perception. Sensations and desires as factors not further analyzable, and feeling as something vague and not yet analyzed, may also have their place in truth, but are not expressions of logical principles. There is a difference between truth as relation or structure and truth as fundamental framework or logical principle. All mental forms may express truth as structure, but only the primary forms seem capable of expressing its fundamental framework. It may of course be said that logical principle has a place in the imagination, but this holds just so far as the content of the imagination is expressed in the primary forms of concept, judgment, etc., and not in the form of concrete images. It would then seem that the only forms in which logical principle gets expressed in consciousness are to be found in concept, judgment, inference, and reasoning.

The logical core and system of relations conditioned by it are then brought to consciousness or massed in mind under the conditions of the primary forms. These forms seem to be of two sorts, concept and inference on the one hand, and on the other judgment and reasoning. Concepts and inferences as mental forms are relatively static and fixed. They stand for the products of thought and are forms which may easily be retained by the mind. In language concepts are generally represented by terms and inferences by propositions. Concepts may express universal relations and are therefore forms appropriate to the expression of the fundamental relations of the logical core. Relations of many features of truth may be conceived by abstraction and generalization from particular details, but logical principles cannot be so conceived, they are brought to mind rather by subtraction of the unessential factors and by the selection and recognition of those factors which form the conditions or *sine qua non* of truth; and it is largely in inferences that the particular details are included under the logical principles. Most important of all is the fact that in concepts and inferences universal relations are grasped and the vast range of the logical principles of the core is brought within the compass of mind. Thus broad perspectives and points of view may be attained.

In contrast with concept and inference, judgment and reasoning are distinctly dynamic and active mental forms or functions. Judgments may be represented in propositions and reasonings in series of propositions, but as reasoning is an extended form of judgment it may be sufficient to consider the character of judgment. Judgments seem to be essentially synthetic in form, that is, in judgments one concept is added to another or is brought to bear on it. It might be better to say that in judgment one term or relation or group of relations is seen to be connected with another term or relation. This moving, synthetic character of judgment makes it possible for the mind to run through long series of relations, to take in larger and larger perspectives by recognizing more fundamental relations, and so to overcome the more static grouping of relations in concept. Furthermore, judgment makes it possible for the mind to penetrate and see the connections among the logical principles, and to appreciate the bearings of these principles on the details of the systems of truth; and above all it should be recognized as the mental function which is the basis of all research and pursuit of knowledge. If truth is on the march and moves from stage to stage, it is in judgment that the mind recognizes this movement and itself moves along with it. Judgment as well as concept can be of universal relations and therefore is also capable of expressing the logical principles and the fundamental structure of truth. Both concept and judgment give range to the mind by bringing logical principle to consciousness, but both have their limitations. They are the organs of science and knowledge and between them make possible and limit intellectual work. The unity of the concept is limited by the number of factors which a concept or a conceptual grouping can include. Though any factor in the concept may, as a universal, have extensive range, the limitation of the concept may be partly overcome by judgment and its additions to concept; but judgment may easily become discursive and rambling so that the additions brought about through judgment need to be gathered together again in concept. Thus concept and judgment supplement each other yet together involve limitations to the attainment of knowledge.

It is then in concept and judgment and in their extension in inference and reasoning that truth is brought to and massed in the mind with full consciousness of the structure of truth as based on the logical core of fundamental relations. In regard to this relation of concept and judgment to truth it should not be forgotten that truth with its core is one thing and that the including and massing of truth in concept and judgment is another. Truth in all its relations stands out as primary and independent while the shape it takes in concept and judgment is secondary but no concern of truth itself. Therefore an attempt to base truth or its core on concept or judgment is a mistake. A psychology of truth or knowledge cannot be the basis of a theory of truth or knowledge or the basis of logic.

It is a common view of truth that it is an idea or concept with objective reference. According to this view, truth implies the relation of the idea of the concept to the object and therefore it is grounded in part in concept. Such a view is an expression of the correspondence conception of truth. One reason that the mind easily accepts it is to be found in its use of symbols, particularly linguistic symbols. A word may undoubtedly refer to a truth or a relation in the system of truth, and such a word is often more prominent in the mind than the object or relation to which it refers; yet the word does not really represent but only suggests the truth or relation. If the truth or relation were not given to the mind it could never be known. The same holds in part of the image. So far as the image only suggests and does not really represent the truth, it yields no truth, and so far as it embodies the truth it is identical with the truth and is not a representative of it. But that truth is given to consciousness in concept does not mean that it is founded in concept and therefore in mind. If the logical principles are called concepts or categories, it should not be understood that they are to be regarded as mental principles. They are not products of the mind but relevant to the structure of truth. Mind may not see truth and grasp its full significance as grounded in the logical core without concepts, but this does not mean that logical principles are the products of the concept and of mind. It signifies only that mind without concepts would be blind to the logical core.

The same difficulty is to be found with the view that truth is founded in judgment, and that the logical principles may be deduced from the fundamental forms of judgment. Though the relation of truth and its logical principles may be expressed in judgment, judgment does not determine those relations and principles but only the mode in which they are given in consciousness. Even the variations in the modes of judgment are dependent upon the demands of truth, that is, the different kinds of relations and principles determine the types of judgment needed to express them. That judgments are both quantitative and qualitative is due to quantitative and qualitative relations in the system of truth, and it is not due to any mental character of judgment, for instance, to some phase of the hypothetical judgment, that relations such as causal relations or relations of dependence hold among the relations making up truth. Nor does movement in judgment or its synthetic function of bringing more and more to consciousness offer a basis for the moving structure of truth: it is rather the way in which a changing and growing truth is encompassed within the limited content of mind. The mental character of the expression of truth in judgment has then to do only with the limited grasp of truth in consciousness. Any judgment theory of truth is therefore a misconception of the relation of truth to mind.

Concepts and judgments being mental rather than logical forms and not the basis of a theory of truth, it should be clear that in any account of the relation of mind to the logical core these mental forms must be regarded as the way in which logical principles are massed in consciousness. Of course it may be said that to treat concepts and judgments as mental forms of logical truth is only to state in different words that mind is an awareness-unity of limited truth, except that these mental forms of logical truth are special forms or ways in which consciousness includes truth within its limited content. Under the limitations of perception there is no truth, no group of relations, given to consciousness which can be called logical truth, and under the limitations of imagination much truth is given which is not logical truth. Again, the larger part of concepts and judgments are not of logical or fundamental relations. In fact, most of the relations given to consciousness are not fundamental or basic relations. Concepts are acquired by laying stress upon or attending to certain features or relations in the field of consciousness. These features or relations are selected as significant in the understanding of some problem or in the furthering of some interest or purpose, all irrelevant features being subtracted or left out. The features selected are mostly general characters of the group of relations involved and based in part on perception and imagination, and the experiences of life. As general characters they are not necessarily fundamental principles. But if the purpose of the mind is to find such fundamentals, then by further and more careful selection and by further subtraction of unessentials it may come upon certain features which it recognizes as fundamentals and therefore as logical principles and conditions of truth. This attainment of logical principles by the mind involves great refinement in both concept and judgment, it being not merely a recognition of the fundamentals themselves but also of their relation to truth as its condition. It should be clear, however, on the one hand, that concepts and judgments as forms in which truth is massed in consciousness are not merely the organs of logical principles but of all universal relations, yet as organs of universal relations they may include fundamental relations; and on the other hand, that it is only in concepts and judgments that the logical core can be brought to consciousness.

Abstraction is then incidental in bringing logical principles to mind. The essential thing is for the mind to see clearly the logical principles as forming the formal framework of truth and its various systems. This formal framework is synthetic; it is the basis of unity and connection in the systems of truth. It unifies and connects in the sense that it supplies the various kinds of relations needed to give unity and ground to the special and more detailed relations of the systems. But as synthetic it does not play the role merely of a static unity of truth but also as the basis of truth's progress and movement from stage to stage. In fact, it may itself change as with the development of the systems of truth finer and more perfect logical principles are required. The formal framework offers a basis for both static and dynamic syntheses.

The relation of the framework to the mind may possibly be made clearer by reference to synthesis and analysis. Most logicians and psychologists would say that analysis and synthesis represent complementary functions. The question as to the relative value of analysis and synthesis depends on whether they are considered from the point of view of truth or of the mind. For truth, synthesis is supreme and analysis subsidiary. As composed of relations, truth is by its very nature connective and therefore synthetic. To break it up by analysis would be to destroy its structure. Analysis may appear in truth as it progresses from stage to stage. In a stage of truth certain relations of a prior stage may be discarded and such relations may be said to be broken up or disrupted. If this procedure be regarded as analysis, then it is analysis incidental to and preparatory to a better synthesis. Logic is essentially the science of the fundamental conditions of synthesis; it is not a science of analysis taken either as a science of tautology or of disruption. From the point of view of mind, however, the situation is different. In its activity to discover truth and logical principle it analyzes and separates and also synthesizes and connects the various factors and features of truth which fall within its content. Synthesis and analysis might here seem to go together, as indeed they do as mental functions. If the mind is after truth or specific items of truth it may be as much concerned with breaking up and analyzing its content as with putting it together in syntheses. It depends upon the kind of relations it is seeking. But if the mind is intent upon attaining logical principle, then its synthetic activity becomes a primary activity and its analytical activity a secondary one. Analytic logic is inadequate; it is a kind of mental logic or aid to the mind in grouping and separating its concepts rather than a genuine logic of truth. The mind may separate and connect *ad libitum*, but truth in its structure is connected. The principles of identity and difference, as also the principle of contradiction, which have been regarded as the bulwarks of analytic logic, are principles of synthesis as well as of analysis. Logic may then be mental in the sense that it implies the recognition of the fundamental syntheses of truth on the part of the mind. But the processes of analysis and synthesis are mental in a sense that they are due to the limitations of the mind. Attention, discrimination, selection, and the contracted recognition of principles of truth are mental functions made necessary by the limited content of consciousness. If the mind could take in all truth in one great intuition then these mental functions would not be necessary, but the mind being what it is, taking in only limited content, it is only through such functions that it can know truth and its formal framework, and it falls to psychology to understand and elucidate these functions.

The value of the formal framework of truth, of its logical core, together with the mental functions involved in grasping it, lies in the great range of truth and systems of truth which the formal framework and mental functions bring within the compass of consciousness. The content of the mind is lacking in any high degree of concreteness. There is awareness and unity of relatively few factors as content, but if principles are included among those factors those principles may define and condition large spheres of truth and so bring the mind in contact with extensive systems. The mind thus has the key to most systems and objects of truth, possibly to all, at least in form.

Reference has already been made to the freedom of truth as relative to the mind, but now cognizance should be taken of the freedom of the mind relative to truth. The mental forms of concept and judgment and of the processes of analyzing and synthesizing on the part of the mind make it possible for the mind to roam all about in the realm of truth. To be sure, vast concretions cannot be attained; but insight into the form and principle of things is possible. In bringing truth and objects within its content, the mind is not limited to perception and to the happenings of the present. It may have thoughts of the past and of the future, and again of systems which are not temporal in character. The span of imagination, the span of consciousness which goes beyond the present, would have little significance if it were not for concept and judgment. Images without concepts and judgments would be mere repetitions of perception and feeling. Mind is limited only by the limitations of concepts and judgments in their power to bring the framework of truth to mind, and by the range of the imagination.

It is important to note in this connection that the freedom of mind with respect to truth means that truth, any and all truth, may condition mind and not that mind is conditioned by some particular system of truth. The framework of truth is opened to it and its content may come from and belong to any part of truth. Therefore the content of consciousness is not necessarily in time and its sequences are not necessarily temporal.

The study of the relation of mind to the logical framework or core has now been shown to be largely a study of the way in which concept and judgment as mental forms are related to the logical framework. They are the forms which the limited mind uses in bringing the principles of the core within its content. Before the relation of psychology to physical science is taken up, it might be appropriate to show how these forms are connected with the kinds of limitation noted above. Concept and judgment are affected chiefly by the first two kinds of limitation, limitation due to the span of consciousness and that due to the change of content in consciousness. In a concept or form embodying a universal, consciousness tries, so to speak, to reach out beyond itself; but because of its limited span it is obliged to leave out most of the particulars which fall under the universal. Any change in the content may bring more particulars under the concept, but those at first included may then disappear. The range of the concept remains largely formal. So also with judgment. While it might seem that the natural movement of judgment could make up for the more static character of concept, it is still true that as the mind moves from judgment to judgment the earlier judgments fall out of consciousness so that later judgments do not include all the judgments which have led up to them. Limitation with respect to the division of the factors in the content of consciousness may affect both concept and judgment, mostly in activities where analysis is involved; and limitation relative to the individual consciousness may affect the application of the concept to various fields to which it applies; but these two kinds of limitation are of less consequence where the logical core is concerned. It is for psychology, the psychology of the logical, to work out the forms and to reconstruct the pattern in accordance with which logical framework is brought within the limitations of consciousness. With the bare outline and suggestions here given as to the psychological truth to be added to objective truth, the relation of psychology to physical science may now be considered.

Consideration of the relation of psychology to physical science means consideration of the objects of these branches of science as relative to each other. The objects of both branches are real objects, objects which lay claim to existence as distinct from imaginary objects or objects which ought to be. The object of psychology has already been outlined and its essential characteristics defined. The object of physical science may probably be most simply defined as the world of space–time including all that is contained within it. It is the system studied by mechanics, physics, astronomy, chemistry, geology, and biology, and it includes substances, stars, electrons, light, energy, organisms, etc. It is concerned with the laws, arrangement, and sequence of the contents of space–time, the changing empirical world. It might be claimed today by some that space–time is relative to and dependent on light, energy, electrons, or other more fundamental objects, and that therefore it is not the primary determinant of the physical world; but for purposes of definition and demarcation, particularly where the relation of the physical world to the mental is concerned, space–time is sufficiently clear as a criterion and not likely to lead to confusion. The physical world may then be regarded as the space–time world, the world of temporal change as known to consciousness and as entering into the content of consciousness but still as distinct from consciousness in the sense that it is not inclusive of consciousness or mind.

Now it should be noted on the one hand, as the laws of the physical system are largely mechanical, that they are dependent on mathematical principles and these again on logical principles, so that physical science is dependent on mathematics and logic. The space–time system of physical science is largely a spatio-temporal plan or map plus equations expressing the laws or functions of the relations of the various parts of the plan, and a plan and equations clearly fall within the sphere of mathematical and logical relations. On the other hand, the space–time system is very complex, including many bodies such as chemical substances and organisms. These bodies function in accordance with logical mathematical physical law. It is claimed by some that organisms as distinct from chemical substances involve teleological principles, but however this may be organisms are also dependent upon mechanical law. Then, again, mind seems in many ways to be dependent on the organism, or at least on that part of the organism which is known as the nervous system. Therefore, whether it is regarded as part of the physical system or not, it might be said to be dependent upon the nervous system in a way similar to that in which the organism is dependent upon the inorganic physical world. The mind would then be conditioned by the logical, mathematical, physical, and organic relations. The sequence of the sciences so far as their dependence on one another goes seems to run in a straight line, but the further suggestion has been made that logical principles as forms of knowledge are dependent on the mind and that logic is in a way dependent on psychology. If this suggestion be taken seriously the various branches of truth form a circle. Such a circle of knowledge or truth would mean that any particular branch of knowledge would condition itself and be conditioned by itself. For instance, organisms would condition the mental world, which would condition the logical, mathematical, and physical worlds and so include the organisms which would be conditions of themselves. This circle of knowledge is of course impossible, but to suggest it has a value in that it opens up the question where the circle may be broken — whether in one place or in more than one place.

If the circle is taken as that of physics, biology, psychology, logic, mathematics, and back to physics again, there would seem to be four places where a break might possibly come. It might first of all be said to be between mathematics and physics. If the break were made here and the rest of the circle kept intact, the world of physical science would be primary, and through biology and psychology it would be the basis of logic and mathematics; the result would be a kind of materialism. But quite apart from any such consequence it should not be forgotten that physical science would be lost without mathematics. Physical truth is very dependent upon mathematical truth and closely interwoven with it. It would be difficult to think of a physical science which was not a mathematical physical science. Of course it may be said that mathematical truth is more universal than physical truth in the sense that it conditions other systems beside the space–time system, but its being the condition of other systems does not prevent it from being the condition of the physical system. Then, if it should be said that mathematics pursues an *a priori* method and physics pursues an empirical method, it should be remembered that the method of hypothesis in physical science is not essentially different from the postulational method used in mathematics. On the whole it would seem about impossible to break the continuity between mathematics and physical science, therefore the break in the circle is probably not to be made at this point.

In the second place, it might be suggested that the break could come between physics and biology, between the inorganic and the organic spheres. The only reason for making the break here would seem to be that the organic sphere is thought to involve teleological principles and the inorganic sphere not to need such principles. Though teleological principle is more noticeable and more useful in understanding organisms than is the case with the inorganic, still the inorganic sphere may be understood teleologically. The solar system, a molecule, or a pure mathematical system may be conceived of teleologically, that is, from the point of view of the whole rather than from the point of view of the units which compose the whole. Therefore if the organic sphere cannot be explained without teleological principle it would seem probable that this teleological principle is continuous with an inorganic teleological principle. In any case there is no good reason for separating the organic from the inorganic. Organisms are true parts of the space–time system, they are subject to its laws and continuous with their inorganic environment. Biology is then dependent on physics fully as much as physics is dependent on mathematics and logic.

In the third place, the break might be said to fall between biology and psychology, between the organic and the mental. Undoubtedly mind is dependent in many ways on the nervous system and so on the organism. It might even seem as if it were related to the organic as the organic is related to the inorganic, or that it were really part of the space–time system. According to behaviorism, mind is regarded as a function in the physical system, and the content theory can hardly avoid regarding mind as in some way physical because it regards the content as in time and that which is in time is also in space. But the theory that beside content mind includes awareness-unity cannot place mind in the space–time world. Not only is awareness-unity not in space–time, but part of the content of awareness-unity is also not in space–time; therefore it would not seem possible to regard mind as entirely dependent on the physical system or as really part of that system. At least there is a partial break between the mental and the organic, mind being more extensive than its organic condition. At most, psychology is then only partly dependent on biology.

Finally, a break might be said to hold between logic and psychology. Most of what has been said in these pages would point in the direction of making logic entirely independent of psychology. The structure of the mind, its activity, and its function do not produce truth or the logical core of truth. The framework of truth is not framed by the mind; it is relative to the details of truth. To know truth may imply mind, but to be truth is to be a structure independent of mind. Logical relations may condition mathematical relations and mathematical relations may condition physical relations and they again in turn through organic relations may in part condition mind, but mind cannot be said to condition logical relations. There is then a true break in the circle of knowledge, between logic and psychology.

Thus the relation of the sciences to one another would seem not to be circular but rather in the form of a straight line, or of a series which does not return upon itself, the various sciences being arranged in order of dependence. If logic were the first member of the series then psychology could be the last, but without complete dependence on biology. The status of psychology would then be left somewhat uncertain. But now it should be noted that although logic is not dependent on psychology, and logical relations are not dependent on mind, mind is dependent on logical relations. Mind is dependent on logical relations directly, though also indirectly, since it is dependent upon the organism and that indirectly on logical relations. The same holds of the relation of mind to mathematical relations and to relations in the space–time system as well as to relations in other systems. In fact, mind may be in direct relation with any sphere of truth, irrespective of its dependence upon the nervous system and the organism. Mind cannot then be treated as dependent on the organism in the same way that the organism may be dependent upon the inorganic and the whole physical system, because it may be immediately related to any phase of truth. Mind is, of course, dependent, but its dependence on truth is not limited to any particular sphere nor confined to dependence on the organic sphere.

If mind is thus not dependent on any particular sphere and is free to roam about in the various regions of truth, it might seem as if it were something quite different from the physical system. Mind may be defined as consciousness and therefore not as a function of the nervous system or as content in time or in space–time, but as something having greater range than the space–time system or anything in that system. And, again, the physical system as the space–time system may be said to be more extensive than mind, in as much as the physical system implies more than is ever penetrated by mind. What is then more natural than to think of mind and the physical world as distinct regions of truth? Yet they are not entirely distinct, because they overlap. Some contents of mind are also temporal and therefore physical, and the mind may know the physical world at least in part. How then are mind and the physical world related or connected? As mind is dependent on truth, to inquire how it is dependent on physical truth would help to bring out its relation to the physical world. It appears to be dependent upon the physical world in two ways: in being conscious of the physical system or any part of it or of any truth about it, mind is dependent on that system, and in so far as it is dependent on the organism or the nervous system, it is in a more specific way dependent. Both kinds of dependence must be considered.

Though mind is not entirely dependent on the physical system, and the physical system is more extensive than mind, mind is dependent on that system in so far as it is conscious of any phase of it; that is, that phase of the physical system is logically prior to the mind's thought of it. The mind thinks it or gathers it up in concepts and to some extent in percepts and feelings, and the way it is so gathered up is a mental addition to it. A law of the physical world would be grasped by the mind in concept or judgment, so also the plan of the solar system or the arrangement of atoms in a molecule. A feather floating through the air might be both perceived and conceived, but any of these objects referred to would have their place first in the space–time system and then as related to awareness-unity. This kind of dependence is general, and like the dependence of the mind on any system of truth it involves the object and the mental condition of conception and all the functions involved in knowing.

The mind may thus roam about in the physical system, gathering up various parts of it and understanding its principles. It does this largely by means of the functions of conception and judgment and may also be helped by perception. Though concept and judgment give breadth, range, and depth to consciousness of the physical system, perception seems always to be a feature of the content of consciousness. Now it should be noted that the perception or the object as perceived is limited to the present in time; more strictly speaking, to the here and now in the space–time system. The mind does not have perceptions of the past, of the future, or of other than present physical objects. It might possibly be said that a perception of the heavens is a perception of objects many of which are perceived as they were at some past time, but, strictly speaking, the perception of the heavens is a perception of the pattern of objects as they affect an organism at a given moment and in a given place. In fact, perception seems to be very closely associated with the organism or with the nervous system, particularly so far as the activity of the sense organs is involved. It may well be that the nervous system conditions the mind so far as it conditions the mind's perceptions. It may be said that the mind is in all respects specifically conditioned by the nervous system and that without a nervous system there would be no mind. But it is important to make certain distinctions at this point.

It might be contended that the mind is merely a direct awareness of some of the activities of the nervous system or of patterns of the brain; and it might also be contended that the mind is a function of the brain and therefore entirely dependent on it. As for the first contention, if all the content of the mind were activities or patterns of the brain, the mind would be limited to the here and now of the brain. There may be such activities and patterns corresponding to the content of the mind and in some ways conditioning it, but if they make up the sole content of the mind it would be impossible to have direct knowledge of the past or of systems other than physical systems. If, as according to the second contention, the mind is a function of the brain it is not necessary to regard it as entirely dependent on the brain. It may be a function of the brain in the sense that it is related to the brain but its relation to the brain would not prevent inclusion in it of content not included in the brain. So far as the mind perceives and uses perceptual imagery it may be here and now, but through concepts, judgments, reasoning, and thoughts expansion beyond the here and now may be very extended.

Should it be said that concepts, judgments, thoughts, etc., merely abstract from perception, and the here and now and are therefore limited to content taken from the physical world, it may be answered that in imaginary systems or in all systems other than the physical system the make-up and organization of such systems is different from that of the physical system. Though many if not all of the features and relations of these systems may have been suggested by factors abstracted from the physical system the composition of these other systems and the principles characteristic of them cannot be regarded as mere offshoots of the physical system, since they form separate and independent syntheses. For instance, the presuppositions and postulates of a moral system together with the moral system itself can hardly be said to be nothing but an activity of the brain. The way out of the difficulty is to recognize on the one hand that perception is of the here and now and is limited to the present, and that so far as the mind is conditioned by the present, whether in perception or in its other functions, it is conditioned by the nervous system; and on the other hand that the mind, though linked with the present, may include in its content relations and systems of relations reaching far beyond the narrow limits of the present and the activities of the nervous system. The mind, therefore, touches the physical system in the present moment of time, and it does so in perception, imagery, and feeling, with a certain degree of concrete detail included in its content. It may also have contact with phases of past time and may look into the future, as it may also conceive of other than temporal systems. One of the great mistakes which psychology, particularly empirical psychology, has made has been to start with or to emphasize the study of sensation and perception, then to go on to imagery and feeling, and finally to take up concept, judgment, and will, as if these latter were pyramided up and depended mainly on sensation and perception. To regard percepts as central to mind and concepts as abstractions or adumbrations of percepts is to distort mind and to throw the content of consciousness out of balance. It would seem reasonable to start with the content of mind in its fullest range and most complete synthesis and then to come down to the details and groups of relations found in the concrete in perception, sensation, and feeling. Just as a sensation may be regarded as an item or factor in perception, so perception may be regarded as an item or bit of concretion, however important, in the whole field of mental content. As it is the work of psychology to determine all the content of mind, a view of the whole of this content should come first, it being easier to determine the detail relatively to the whole than by taking it up piece by piece. The point of view taken in Chapter II is that synthesis comes first and that the value of analysis lies in filling out the synthesis and perfecting it. No psychology is complete which does not conceive mind in its wholeness.

But men live too much in the present to be unbiased in their conception of mind. Perception may seem to occupy the center of the field of consciousness, and perhaps it does generally usurp this position. Yet the true center of the field or content of consciousness is the focal point of attention, the point of greatest clearness and intensity. The focus of attention may include a percept, or a feeling, or an image, or a concept or judgment, or even a relation which cannot be fully expressed in perception or imagery. It is interesting to note that Kant realized, beside perception and memory and over and above constructive imagination, that conception and judgment were necessary to round out the mind. Without them systematic knowledge would be impossible.[5] Much has been said about imageless thought. This does not mean that in the process of thinking no images are ever used, it means only that there are thoughts which do not require images. Just as without percepts and feelings there would be no mind at all, so without images there would be no thoughts or concepts, but at the same time the thoughts and concepts are more than the images and may function without them. In other words, in thoughts and concepts there are relations not fully expressed in images. The range and the expanse of mind exceed not only perceptions but also the reverberations and rearrangements of perceptions in imagination. There is, then, mental content which is more than perception, feeling, imagery, and their products.

So far, in the consideration of the relation of mind to the physical world, mind has been taken largely as consciousness from the point of view of the single awareness-unity of content. It has not been considered from the point of view of the sequence of its content. In the same way that it is possible to refer to stages of truth and stages of positive knowledge it is possible to refer to mental stages. The sequence of mental stages has been generally treated as temporal sequence. It should now be clear why there may be sequence of a sort which is not temporal. In Chapter III reference was made to the view that the mental or psychical is in time only as contrasted with the physical, which is in space as well as in time. This view was set aside because it was pointed out that whatever is in time is also in space and therefore the mental could not be merely temporal. The advocates of this view were not utterly wrong. If they had been asked to point out phenomena which were in time and not in space they would very probably have referred to feelings and thoughts. Now if pleasure is taken as an example of feeling it would seem that it is in space and must be referred to space as well as to time. But the case is different with thoughts. They undoubtedly

[5] Immanuel Kant, *Kritik der reinen Vernunft* (1st ed., Riga, 1781), pp. 98–128.

follow each other in sequence and can also very generally be said not to be in space. If they are not in space they are not in time, but not being in time does not prevent them from being in sequence. It is quite possible to speak of the "stream of consciousness," but this stream does not have to be all a temporal stream. If the content of consciousness changes, one stage of content giving way to another, it may be asked what sort of sequence is involved. It is clear that part of the stream, part of the change, is change in time; but it is equally clear that part of it is non-temporal change. The content of sensations, perceptions, images, feelings, emotions, and the like flows in time, and by its nature and structure is very closely connected with the space–time world, whereas the content of thoughts, concepts, reasoning, memories, ideals, etc., changes and alters but largely not in temporal sequence. This latter kind of content, if judged by its structure, is often a sequence of very varied and diverse objects. From the thought of justice the mind may turn to the contemplation of the plan of a building to be built, then to the concept of a mathematical proposition, then to the memory of something that happened ten years ago, and after that to the consideration of the sale of a lot of land. These contents as objects do not follow each other in temporal sequence. The only reason for regarding them as in temporal sequence is that they are connected in consciousness with content which does change in temporal sequence. The images which serve as a help to thought, the perceptions which run along often in association with concepts, and the general body of feeling which gives a background to the content of consciousness, all emphasize the temporal continuity of the content of the mind. But just because in consciousness images are related to thoughts and percepts to concepts it is not necessary to suppose that the temporal sequence of images and percepts must be carried over to thoughts and concepts. The only reason for regarding the sequence of images, percepts, and feelings as being in time is that they have a proper place in a temporal sequence and in the space–time world, and in the same way the reason for regarding the sequence of thought, concepts, memories, etc., as not in time is that their nature and sequence is such that they do not fit into a time series. It is important, then, to bear in mind that not only is there content of consciousness which is not of the here and now but there is also sequence of content in consciousness which has no true place in time. This type of sequence might be called the sequence of objective content.

The relation of the mental or psychical world to the physical or space–time world would now seem to be that of a kind of half-dependence of the former on the latter. Perceptual objects, images, and feelings have their place in the physical system as functions of the nervous system and they change in time just as the physical system changes in time. As mental functions these functions are therefore dependent on or actually identical with functions of the brain. They are physical primarily because they are determined by their relation to the space–time world, and they are mental secondarily because their inclusion in consciousness is an addition to what they are by virtue of the place they hold in the physical world. As for objects of thought, conceptual objects, memories, and ideals — in so far as they get suggestions from, are assisted by, or make use of perceptual objects, images, and feelings they depend on the nervous system. But they must not be dragged down to the level of perceptual objects, images, etc., nor treated as following in temporal sequence or merely as functions of the nervous system. They also function independently of the brain, and as content of consciousness they include objects and sequences of objects which in their structure are not conditioned by the nervous system. This content may be part of any system or sub-system of truth, and therefore in including truth of one system or another it is free from the conditions of the physical world unless its objective content is part of that world, and even if it does include some part of the physical world such part need not be narrowed down to perceptual objects or objects of the present. In its objective content the mind is just as free to range about in all parts of the physical world as it is to range about in other worlds or systems. So far, however, as the mind does include any part of the physical world in its content, the mind follows the truth of that world. As all truth is primary and inclusion of it in the mind is secondary, physical truth is primary and consciousness of it is secondary. The freedom of truth must be recognized. It is independent and must be determined independently of mind. At the same time there is a freedom of mind, that is, a freedom to roam about in the field of truth. Mind is dependent on the physical world so far as it thinks physical things or includes physical truths in its content, and it is also dependent on the physical system so far as the nervous system specifically conditions some of its functions.

The twofold dependence of the mind on the physical world, together with its independence of that world, having been considered, as also its independence taken both with respect to the mind's objective content and sequence of objective content, something should now be said as to the existence or reality of the mental and physical spheres. In contrast with logical truth as the formal framework of all systems, and in contrast with imaginary systems and teleological systems of truth, mental and physical systems are real, existent, or actual in the sense that they condition and include a detail of relations which in some degree is accessible to mind and determinable in knowledge. Such existent detail might be referred to as phenomena or as phenomenal reality to distinguish it from the ultimate reality or the full concrete framework of truth. The term *experience* might also be used in connection with the detail, and, since experience is an ambiguous term suggesting both the space–time worlds of empirical science and the content of mind as experienced in consciousness, it might be regarded as including both spheres of existence. But just because it is ambiguous it is of little use in distinguishing the two spheres. And furthermore the two spheres overlap. If both systems are accessible to mind and therefore fall within its content they might be thought to be existent so far as they are presented to mind. But *presentation,* like experience, is ambiguous and also does not do justice to the extent of the space–time world. The physical world has been defined as the space–time world. Any detail or bit of phenomena would be physical if it had a place in the space–time system. Now the most concrete part of the space–time world accessible to mind is the present. Any attempt to test or try out an hypothesis with respect to the physical world involves reference to the detail of present events, details here and now. It would therefore seem reasonable to hold that anything is physically existent which is connected with the present or which belongs to the space–time system which includes the present. In knowledge physical existence is tested in the present. From the point of view of truth, the physical world is the space–time world; from the point of view of knowledge and of the mind, physical existence is rather the spatio-temporal extension of the here and now. But now if physical existence radiates from the present the present is not sufficient to express mental existence. Mental content often centers in the past and the future and in systems other than physical. The mentally existent is that which falls within awareness-unity or is given as its content. The term *given*, meaning given in awareness-unity, is more extensive than the term *present* and better suited to suggest mental existence. Anything that is thus given may lay claim to mental existence just as anything which is present or related temporally or spatially to the present may lay claim to physical existence, and that which is both given and present may lay claim to both kinds of existence. However correctly the mental world may be defined as the world of awareness-unity of limited content and the physical world as the space–time world, the more specific criteria of mental and physical existence may be found in the given and in the present.

It might still be objected that all that is here brought out in characterizing mind may be sufficiently accounted for by the brain function and brain pattern. It should be answered, in the first place, that the brain function as well as the pattern are both in space–time and have not the freedom of range which the mind has; and secondly, that the mind includes in its content objects and even sequences of objects which are not brain functions or brain patterns. It is a mistake to suppose that the brain has any direct or immediate relation to objects or phases of objects as consciousness does. Mind is related not only to the nervous system but also to objects, and it is occupied far more with objects than with the nervous system. The best which the brain can offer is some representation of the object but not the original or any part of it. The immediate contact with objects, however limited, the original activity of knowing, is a function of consciousness and not of the nervous system.

Then it may also be objected that it is inconsistent to speak of non-temporal change. It may be said that sequences of objective content are after all temporal sequences, that all alterations in the content of consciousness are temporal alterations, and that therefore all content of consciousness is in time. It may at first seem arbitrary and even artificial to regard sequences, alterations, or changes in the content of consciousness as not being necessarily temporal changes. Yet how would it be possible to refer to changes of content which as content have no place in time and form no part of a temporal system? For instance, in the understanding of a complex mathematical formula or in the working out of the interrelations of moral principles various groups of features follow one another in sequence as content of the mind, so that there may be said to be a before and an after in the given with an implied past and future relative to the given. Although these groups in their sequences involve a before and after as does time, they can hardly be said to form a temporal sequence or to fit into a time system. Even if the sequences of sensations, images, and feelings which accompany them or which appear in the same content with them are temporal sequences, there is no good reason for regarding the sequences of the groups in the mathematical formula or among the moral relations as falling within or partaking of the sequences of the sensations, images, and feelings, any more than there would be reason to regard a mathematical or moral order as having its place in the brain. Temporal matters, too, may be conceived in non-temporal sequence as in the case of the thoughts of events of the day before yesterday following the thoughts of events of yesterday in the content of consciousness. The real difficulty seems to lie in the fact that many trains of thought or changes of content in consciousness have, as such changes of content, no place in the one system of time. Time is generally regarded both as including events which are successive and changing and as including such events in one system; that is, it is both successive and one. If both these characters of time are recognized, then successions or sequences in the content of consciousness which do not belong in the one system of time are, strictly speaking, non-temporal changes. To overlook the singleness of time and to regard anything that is successive or changing as temporal is to treat time as a general concept inclusive of all sequences. To treat it so is to do violence to time as a unifying conception and as the basis of the physical world as the space–time system. It seems, therefore, wiser to refer to sequences in the content of consciousness which fall outside the system of time as sequences of objective content, and then to regard only those sequences as temporal sequences which have a place in the one time system.

If psychology is the study of the objective as relative to mind, it ought now to be clear how the physical world as objective is relative to mind. Except for the special relation of the nervous system to the mind, the physical system is related to mind very much as other systems of truth are related to it; and the principles, laws, and general outline of the physical world, like logical principles, are massed in consciousness in concept and judgment. But because of the special relation of the nervous system to the mind, the physical system conditions the mind's temporal content and therefore is of great importance in any study of mind.

Now as to the consideration of the relation of the moral system to the mind, of ethics to psychology. It should be noted at once that the moral system is of equal importance with the physical system. It is a system relative to the self-direction of the mind, and like the physical system it is both a system with positive content and also intimately related to the temporal content of mind. It is very easy to think of morality as connected with the activity of mind and therefore to think of the moral system as purely mental, but it should be remembered that the moral system is a system with a structure of its own which cannot be defined on the basis of any mental principle.

A moral system may be said to be first of all a system of ends, purposes, or ideals. It must be distinguished from matters of technique or of means. Though the consideration of the means and technique to realize ends is important, the moral system is primarily a system of ends, and only in a secondary way involves or includes means. Furthermore, as a system of ends it is not concerned with the specific ends themselves but with these ends as interrelated in one whole system. The moral system is then a synthesis or synthetic unity of ends, an ordered system of ends. The unity or order is essential to it. But the ordered system by itself would not be sufficient to make up a true moral system if its relation to the will were not included. Wills or self-directing centers are intimately bound up with the ends and ideals toward which they strive, and the ends and ideals have moral value as ends and purposes of wills. A moral system is therefore not only a system of ends but a system of wills or a system of ends to be willed or of wills directed toward ends.

The moral problem might be suggested by the question, *What ought I?* And this question may be divided into *What ought?* and *Ought I?* *What ought?* suggests the problem of the end or of ends as distinct from means and the central problem of ends is the problem of what *system* of ends ought to be. But such a system does not mean a mere collection of ends having intrinsic value, such as objects of beauty or other objects desired for their own sake. Specific ends, no matter how good or valuable they might be in themselves, have no moral significance, and if all intrinsic value could be realized there would be no moral problem. The moral system first appears as the unity, order, or system of ends which it is possible to realize, and the chief work of moral philosophy has been an attempt to find the principle or principles of that system.

Pleasure has been suggested as the key to the principle of the moral system. As the attainment of any end is usually accompanied by pleasure, hedonists hold that "the greatest possible pleasure" or "the greatest pleasure for the greatest number" is the unifying principle of the moral order. But just because pleasure attaches to specific ends it is not fitted to be used as a principle of order of those ends. Such qualifications as "greatest," or "greatest possible," or "for the greatest number," are generally added to pleasure to make it systematic. Since these qualifications refer to order and imply relations of order it would be more appropriate to apply them to the ends directly, leaving the pleasure which comes with the attainment of ends out of account. Though pleasure may add to the value of ends, it is not central to them, nor is it fitted to give them order or organization. Pleasure would then seem to offer no basis for a moral principle.

In the same way "self-realization," or the fullest possible realization of desires, inclinations, interests, or purposes, has been suggested as a moral principle. Not the emotional result, but the desires, inclinations, etc., as expressions of human nature, are made fundamental. But a similar difficulty appears. Desires, inclinations, etc., are after all ends, and thinking of them as expressions of human nature is merely calling attention to their roots. However much this reference may enhance their intrinsic value it adds nothing to their moral value. And even as ends they have no moral value when taken alone. To have a place in the moral system they must be considered in relation to order. Now the fullest possible realization of ends implies both order and ends. If the order is for the sake of the ends, that is, a means for the fullest and most complete realization of the ends, then the system can hardly be called a moral system. But if the order is a unity or system of ends having value as such a unity and system in its own right, and not as subservient to the ends, it is a genuine moral system. Such a unity of ends means the inclusion of all ends or of all relations of ends to one another within a system of law and order. It is, then, only in the relations among ends, with the ends as terms of the relations, that a moral problem is involved, the moral system being the synthesis of all such relation. In the law and order of the moral system, the law need not mean a universal repetition of the same relation or relations, because the order may well be a progressive order. The universality of a moral system need only mean the totality of the relations, not the sameness of the relations. If the moral system is to be regarded as an end it is different from other ends because it is the end of all ends, and as the unity and form of all ends it is an infinite or never-ending end.

Both "the greatest possible pleasure" and "the greatest possible realization" include order, but the order is other than pleasure or desire. The order would seem to be an order of a vast system of relations as an ideal to be realized but one which can never be completed. It is a formal framework, and the moral life consists in filling in the detail, both in knowledge and by realization in life. The system is an order of orders and these orders are always tentative; just as in the physical system the laws and the details of relations in the stages of realization are never final. It is, therefore, difficult to formulate any moral rules or precepts with any degree of universality, and their formulation is particularly difficult if the moral system is considered as a system of ends without reference to wills or self-directing centers. To answer the question *What ought?* is not sufficient unless the question *Ought I?* is added. *What ought I?* suggests the relation of ends to the will, and in the complete moral system the relation of the order of ends to self-directing centers.

As ends are the expression of wills, so the system of ends or moral order is an expression of wills. Therefore the moral order in the fullest sense is a system of wills willing the synthesis of all ends, or a synthesis of all wills willing an order of ends. The moral world is then a synthesis or system of wills so far as they are directed toward an ideal order. Besides the unity of ends there is a unity of wills, and the wills or self-directing centers making up this unity are themselves ends and form a kind of system of ends; that is, the wills as determined by ends and as being the centers in which ends are effective may be regarded themselves as ends. As such ends they form the true units of a moral system. In fact it would be difficult to give shape to a moral system without treating wills as ends. For an order of ends taken apart from the will is difficult to define. Though certain specific types of ends may be outlined, the development of these ends and the changes in the relation of the ends to one another make it almost impossible to define a moral order of ends. A certain balance in the relation of the ends to one another, justice to all interest, continuity of ideals, etc., may be insisted upon; but as the moral order of ends is an infinite order it is vague and hard to define and it remains always an *x* to be determined. In contrast with an ideal system taken apart from wills, a system of wills is more fundamental and definite.

The moral universe would then seem to consist of all wills or self-directing centers as relative to one another. They would of course be concerned with the system of ends and its realization, with the transforming of the ideal into the real. But moral relations or principles would attach primarily to the system of wills, to the relation of wills in connection with their function of transforming the ideal into the real. In fact, moral precepts are concerned largely with conduct. Moral conduct is the activity of one will relative to and in consideration of the activities of other wills, or the activity of one will with respect to other of its own activities. As Kant says in the first sentence of the first section of the "Foundation of the Metaphysic of Morals," nothing can be thought of as good "absolutely" except a "good will."[6] Morality centers in the will, and the good will is the will which acts consistently with and in harmony with other wills. The synthesis of wills as self-directing and transforming centers acting in harmony with one another as such centers makes up the moral world. The systematization and unification of wills as they make real the ideal is the object of the science of ethics, the great human science.

It is now possible to consider the relation of the moral system to consciousness. The moral system is related to consciousness in two ways, by being known and by affecting the mind's activity. If the moral system is a system of truth

[6] Immanuel Kant, *Grundlegung zur Metaphysik der Sitten* (Riga, 1785).

giving foundation and unity to all ends and wills through the unity of wills, then this system may be known to the mind just as any system of truth is known, and, again, it may be used by the mind as a guide to action. According to the psychologists, will involves idea plus act based upon idea, the idea being an ideal to be realized in or through the act. If the idea includes the moral system or some phase of it and the act follows the idea then the act is a moral act. Both idea and act are essential. Taken together they are related to the moral system very much as in physical science perception is related to the space–time system. Just as the physical or space–time system includes perception, so the moral system includes the moral idea and act. Of course many ideas and acts are not primarily concerned with the moral system, as, for instance, the ideas and acts of an artist in painting a picture, or of a scientist in seeking knowledge; and many ideas and acts fall short of the moral ideal, as is the case with immoral ideas and acts; but all ideas and acts are relevant to the moral system and fall in some degree within its scope. The moral system is the one all-inclusive teleological system and includes all wills whatever their ends or purposes may be.

The moral system as known by the mind, as grasped in idea, is a form of truth, and is therefore brought within the limits of awareness-unity in concept and judgment. It is a formal framework often vaguely conceived which can be filled in gradually. The mind may advance stage by stage in moral truth by means of judgment and reasoning, and it may grasp its moral truth in concept and in inference. But now, as the moral system is primarily non-temporal or super-temporal, and as awareness-unity may include a super-temporal content, knowledge of the moral system or the idea of any stage or phase of it may be super-temporal and therefore not determined by the space–time system. In other words any moral principle or ideal as given in idea or in consciousness may have a non-temporal structure and may be unaffected by temporal events although it may itself condition acts of will which are effective in time. The will as expressing moral truth in idea is then free, that is, free from the temporal process and from the past. This is one way in which it may be said that the will is free, and it is probably the only way in which its freedom has moral significance.

The selective character of the will ought here to be mentioned. If moral truth appears in the mind under the forms of concept and judgment, it should be noted that the will fills in the moral framework by selecting from among the various possibilities of action which appear. Were knowledge complete and were the mind such that it could include in concept all moral truth, then selection would not be necessary. But because the mind is limited, and grasps only one stage of truth with various possibilities for further development, selection is an important function, and it is a function of the will which results from the mind's limitation, from the limitation of its imaginative span. The will may select in accordance with a moral principle or in accordance with some partial perspective; and its virtue would seem to depend upon the range and penetration of its idea or ideas.

But the will is act as well as idea. The act as distinct from the idea takes place in space–time, and it may follow the idea which embodies an ideal or principle which is non-temporal, yet it may itself take place in the time series. As an event in the space–time system it may take place to some degree spontaneously and may not be fully determined by the space–time system. If such indeterminism is true, then the act may be said to be in some sense free, and as a result the will may be said to be free but in an entirely different way from the way mentioned in the foregoing paragraph in which the will was said to be free through idea. The freedom of the act in the physical system would seem to have no moral value as does the freedom through the idea.

In addition to this consideration of freedom it is important to note that the will is effective only in time and again only in the present. So far as knowledge is concerned, the will may penetrate into all corners of the super-temporal, but if it is to bring about anything or to change the world in any respect it must initiate its activity in the present. The past, of course, it cannot change and any effect it may have upon the future can only be brought about by influencing the present. If will is content of awareness-unity its limitation is twofold. As idea it is limited by the given, that is, only as the full range of content is limited; and as act it is limited to that part of the given which is known as present time. Because of this double character in its limitation it is possible for the will to transform the ideal into the real.

The moral system as a system of wills, willing ends, and as the most comprehensive teleological system, stands in relation to the mind very much as the physical system does. In the first place it is objective. It is a system of truth like the physical system. It is inclusive of all ends and purposes just as the space–time system is inclusive of all that is in space and time. It may be thought of as ideal rather than as real but it is nevertheless all-inclusive in its sphere. Secondly, it is related to the present. It is inclusive of present acts as the space–time system is inclusive of present perceptions. If the relation to the present were left out in either system that system would be a purely imaginary system. Thirdly, both systems determine the present and are thus effective in the world. The space–time system conditions the present mechanically or otherwise and the moral system conditions the present teleologically and by determining what it ought to be. Though the physical system seems to express only an *is* and the moral system expresses an *ought,* both are systems of determining conditions.

The objective character of these two systems, the moral and the physical, which in some way include and determine the present is of the greatest importance. If the objective order of truth is primary and its massing in consciousness secondary, and if the objective order is necessary in order that the mental order be determined, then those two most fundamental orders, the physical and the moral, are crucial in determining mind. The distinction, for instance, in the physical system between the present, the past, and the future makes possible the mental distinction between perception, memory, and imagination; and the distinction between space or order in perception and the detail falling within the order makes possible the distinction between the order of sensation and sensation itself. In the moral system, the distinction between the order of ends and the ends makes possible the distinction within the will between ideal and desire, and the distinction between idea and act forms the basis for the two types of virtue, wisdom and self-control. Not only do fundamental mental factors come to light through reconstruction based on these two fundamental objective orders, but each of these orders prevents the mind from being absorbed in the other order. The two orders seem to cross or to come to a focus in the present moment, yet the physical present does not fully absorb the will, nor does the moral present — the act — take up or include the full physical present. Apart from the larger sphere of the given in consciousness, and irrespective of imaginary systems and the aesthetic world, the present in the content of consciousness is not fully accounted for in either physical or moral terms. As the moral and physical systems seem not to form one system in the world of truth, the mind is dependent on at least two sources for its determination.

Granted, now, that the content of mind is limited truth massed in various ways in consciousness, and that this content consists of relations belonging to various systems of truth, including the physical and moral systems, two questions arise. In the first place it may be asked if the various systems, and principally the physical and moral systems, in any way form one system of truth. Is there any ultimate unity to truth which as given in consciousness appears to come from different objective orders and sources? And in the second place it may be asked whether the mind has any bearing on the possible ultimate unity of truth. Though it seems to be secondary to and dependent on the objective orders does it by any chance give a clue to the nature of the ultimate order? The whole matter may be stated in another way. The logical core is the formal unity of all truth, the condition or conditions of all relations and of the various systems of relations; but now is there a material unity of truth, a concrete system or ultimate object including all relations? Can all systems of relations be embraced within one concrete whole or system? And if there be such a system what place would the mind have in that system? Would it be essential to that concrete whole, or only an unimportant detail in the whole? To answer these questions the ontological problem and its relation to mind must be considered.

The ontological problem is here referred to as the problem of the ultimate framework of truth, while in Chapter II it was referred to as the problem of the ultimate framework of reality. The reason for referring to truth instead of reality is that the demand for totality or the implication of an ultimate concretion seems to lie in the nature of truth. But owing to the difficulty of uniting all truth in one concrete whole, all systems in one super-system, ontology has generally been confined to the problem of ultimate reality; and if other than real systems of truth have been included they have been regarded as in some way phases of reality. The problem will be taken up both as a problem of truth and as a problem of reality, but as truth is more inclusive than reality the problem will be considered first as a problem of truth.

Truth is synthetic and connected, it is made up of relations and all relations belong to it. It is centered in a logical core, a group of fundamental relations. As all relations in all their connections with one another fall under these fundamental relations, it is natural to ask whether these fundamental relations form the basis for a vast or inclusive system of relations; and even if there are various sub-systems of truth it may still be asked if these systems may not be united in one super-system. The problem is the result of the logical demand for totality, for the unity of all detail under one group of principles. It is based upon the structure of truth.

The possibility of one ultimate system of truth cannot be denied, but neither can it be affirmed. With all the detail and order of relations, with all that is possible and compossible, it is difficult to see how all relations can hang together so as to form one system of truth. The various strata or systems of truth cannot easily be fitted into one another although they often intersect. For instance, the physical system of what is in space–time can hardly be united with the moral system of what ought to be, nor could either one of them be thought of as the basis of the other. The logical core may condition all relations and it may prescribe order to the relations, but the order may be merely the principle of order, that is, order among all relations and in all systems of relations, not necessarily one single order. A minimum of unity is sufficient to satisfy the logical demand for unity. It is possible to speculate as to the ultimate framework of truth and to offer hypotheses as to its unity in one super-system, but so far as the logical unity goes ultimate truth may consist of a collection of systems loosely bound together. In other words, the formal unity of the core offers no clue to the material unity of the whole.

The ontological problem may also be stated not as the demand for the totality of all truth under certain fundamentals but as a result of a progress of truth from stage to stage. Just as the factor of direction in relation leads on to further relations, so one stage of truth leads on to further stages. As each stage tends to be more comprehensive than previous stages it may well be asked if there is not a final all-inclusive stage, a complete system of all truth. Such a stage may lie far beyond all present systems of knowledge and its nature may be incomprehensible, yet ontologists have raised the problem as to the possibility of such a stage and have thought that it might be possible to have a glimmering of its nature.

A final concretion of all relations, a last stage of truth and knowledge, involves the conception of the completion of that which appears incapable of completion. The procedure of truth and knowledge from stage to stage offers no clue as to the nature of a final stage or as to whether there is such a final stage. Though any stage may be more comprehensive than a previous stage it also raises new problems; and a supposedly final stage would seem to point to a still further stage. Not only does the *abc* of knowledge grow, but the *x* of knowledge also grows. The more truth is determined the more there remains to be determined. Metaphysicians like to think of an absolute totality of truth which knowledge approaches step by step. Such an absolute totality would presumably be made up of an infinite variety of relations and the approach to it by stages would involve an infinite progress so that the absolute truth could never be reached. The only accessible truth is the truth of stages. Absolute truth is therefore an enigma. At best it is on a plane with imaginary systems of truth. It cannot be denied, but for knowledge it has only a negative value.

The problem of the ultimate framework of truth can neither be solved by considering its systematic composition nor by treating it as the goal of accessible or determinable truth. The study of it as an ultimate object, system, or concretion yields no result. One other method of attack remains, and this refers to the relation of the ultimate framework of truth to mind. As various systems of truth are accessible to mind it might be suggested that the ultimate framework of truth is given to some ultimate or absolute mind. That mind can roam about through various regions of truth might make it seem fit to be a unifying principle of truth and therefore capable of grasping and connecting all truth in one concrete whole. A mind grasping such a concrete whole would be a super-mind, a mind to which all relations, all systems, and all stages of truth would be given. Is there any evidence for such a mind?

In the analysis of mind made in Chapter II four fundamental features were brought out. These were unity, awareness, content, and the limitation of content relative to unity and awareness. If a super-mind is to be regarded as mind it ought in some way to embody these features. No doubt the vast totality of relations which make up the ultimate framework would form the content of such a super-mind; and the unity of that content, whatever form it might be thought to take, could be regarded as the unity of the super-mind. The sum total of truth would then be spoken of as a mind because it would be a unity or grouping of content. As for the limitation of content, it would hardly apply to a super-mind because the content of the super-mind would include all relations and therefore would be unlimited. Awareness would also seem to have no proper place in the ultimate framework. It may be argued that consciousness is the most perfect expression of a unifying principle, and as the totality of truth implies such a unifying principle it implies consciousness. As consciousness includes awareness as well as unity, awareness is introduced into the ultimate framework. This framework would then be an awareness-unity of all content and therefore an unlimited mind. But awareness of the ultimate framework is by no means implied by it. Royce's attempt to show the possibility of a "presented infinite totality" [7] is superfluous, because the "infinite totality" does not need to be "presented." If awareness is excluded it would hardly be appropriate to speak of the "infinite totality" as "presented" to unity. Furthermore, the function of awareness as distinguishing content from non-content would have no place in the ultimate framework because there is no non-content relative to that framework. A fundamental error in the conception of the super-mind lies in the failure to distinguish the logical unity or the synthetic unity of all truth from the conscious unity. Synthetic unity of all truth there is — without it there could be no truth; but synthetic unity does not carry awareness-unity with it. And synthetic unity of all truth can hardly be called mind; the minimum of mind would seem to imply all four of the fundamental features.

Since the unity of all truth, whether it be a loose or compact unity, does not imply the conscious unity of all truth, there would seem to be no ground for the acceptance of the hypothesis of a super-mind. Mind would seem to give no clue to the ultimate framework of truth. The argument may be stated in a somewhat different way, however. It may be said that the various stages of knowledge are hypotheses constructed by the mind. Then it may be asked what sort of mind could construct systems of truth as found in the various stages of knowledge. And the answer may be made that no individual mind could construct such systems, and therefore a super-mind inclusive of all individual minds would have to be

[7] Royce, *The World and The Individual*, I, 583; see also p. 585.

assumed. This argument for the super-mind is again unsatisfactory. It is true that the systems of truth and knowledge in the various stages are bound up with assumptions, hypotheses, theories, etc., but these so-called constructions are valid because they fit into the structure of truth. Now the structure of truth, however it may alter in the progress from stage to stage, is not constructed by the mind in the sense that it is made, or created, or willed by it. The structure of truth is independent of mind and not its product, therefore it is not possible to assume that mind, whether individual or super-individual, is the condition of truth. Truth stands on its own feet as a vast range of interrelated relations, and the various stages of truth cannot be construed as mental stages. Mind has access to truth and may select that truth which it chooses to contemplate, but it cannot construct truth *ad libitum*.

So much for the consideration of the ontological problem as the problem of ultimate truth. Now as to its consideration as the problem of reality. It is usual to regard the space–time system and mind, the physical world and the mental world, as obviously real or existent. Mind as including immediately given content could hardly be denied existence. The physical world is regarded as real because as a vast dynamic system it conditions all those phases of the mind which are bound up with present time. Imaginary systems are generally treated as non-existent, although so far as they condition mind's knowledge of them they might be said to share in the existence of mind. As for the teleological systems, to the extent to which they express what ought to be rather than what is they are not treated as real, but it would not be unreasonable to allow them a measure of reality so far as they are actually realized in the mental or physical worlds. No doubt the moral world has a very direct bearing on the real world, but in order to be directive of the real world it must lie beyond it and form in part a separate sphere. But if it be granted now that the physical and mental worlds are in any case genuinely real can any suggestion be gotten from them as to ultimate reality?

The physical world contains nothing in its nature to suggest that it is ultimately real. As an elaborate dynamic system pivoted in present time it is far from being a finished or ultimate system. Present time is not complete without past and future time. Past time seems to be gone, and from the point of view of the present not to be real, yet possibly it might be reckoned as a product of the present and therefore belonging to the real. The future is not yet determined and is therefore, strictly speaking, not real or not yet real. The extent of the physical world is also undetermined; it may be limited or unlimited. And with regard to research into its composition no ultimate element has been determined as yet with any certainty. At best, the physical system is an imperfect map plus various laws as to its functioning which may be altered as knowledge advances. Internally, then, it is nothing ultimate; but if it should now be claimed that it is the most real system known, and therefore the sphere in which ultimate reality is eventually to be found, it should be pointed out that the mental world cannot be reduced to the physical. Much is given to mind or consciousness which is not included in the physical system.

If the physical world has nothing to offer toward the solution of the problem of ultimate reality, the mental world can do no better. Should it be said that, because mind can move about in many regions of truth and reality, it probably expresses the ultimate principle of the real, it should not be forgotten that a large part of the physical world is never included in mind. To get around this difficulty it might be said that the physical world includes a mental principle, a sort of mind of nature. This mind might be regarded as analogous to the time-span in perception; it might be said that there is a mind in nature which takes in all its activity in a kind of conscious span. This would bring all present nature within a mind. Possibly this time-span might include the past with the present, but not of course the future, as that is not yet determined. Or again it might be said, as the pan-psychists have said, that nature is replete with a mass of miniature minds. Neither of these suggestions has any real foundation in knowledge of the physical or mental world. Both the idea of a mind in nature and the idea of a system of rudimentary minds are based upon an erroneous conception of mind and of its importance in the real world. That mind can be in tune with truth and reality is no ground for regarding it as anything ultimate. Neither the physical world nor the mental world can suggest anything as to the nature of the ultimate object of reference, whether that object be considered as ultimate truth or reality.

The ontological problem seems then to be insoluble. Hypotheses as to the ultimate framework of truth or reality may be made but no such hypotheses can be verified on the basis of accessible truth or knowledge. It is not even possible to find in mind a suggestion as to the nature of the ultimate object. The ontological problem remains a problem. It can never lead to a system of truth but is rather a question relative to and suggested by the logical core and the various accessible systems of truth, a question as to an object which is inscrutable, an absolute *x*. Thus the study of the ontological problem in connection with the conception of mind yields only negative results, throwing little light on the nature of ultimate reality. And in its turn mind receives no help in its determination from the ultimate object. Mind can be reconstructed on the basis of the physical and moral systems as well as on the basis of other accessible systems, but not on the basis of any ontological system. Psychology and ontology have little in common.

In this chapter, mind and truth have been considered both with respect to the relation of truth to mind and with respect to the place of mind in truth. Psychology was shown to be the science of mind as the massing and grouping of truth in consciousness, mind being truth within the limits of awareness-unity; and it was shown that truth as given to mind was more extensive than present content and that the alterations of the given were not necessarily temporal changes. After consideration of the various forms of limitation of truth in consciousness, the dependence of consciousness or mind on truth and the consequent dependence of psychology on the objective sciences was made clear. Then the relation of psychology to logic, physical science, ethics, and ontology was taken up. The determination of the mind was shown to be dependent on the logical core, the physical world, and the moral world, but not on any ultimate truth or reality. With the relation of mind to truth in its various spheres outlined, a more adequate account of mental truth or of mind as the object of psychological study can now be given.

CHAPTER V

THE SCIENCE OF PSYCHOLOGY

BEFORE THE THEORY OF MIND developed in this work is rounded out it may be well to ask, what is the *x* of psychology? To make clear what is meant by the *x*, reference must be made to mind, to the problem of psychology, and to the correlative of the *x*, the *abc*. If mind is the object or field of psychological investigation, the problem of psychology is to determine the detail of that field. To determine the detail of that field means first to determine in what way and along what lines the determination of that field is to be effected. The lines of determination and the methods to be used must be relative to the general outline of the field to be investigated, mind. In fact no reference could be made to the field without at least some outline of it. This outline is suggested in the definition of mind as awareness-unity of limited content and in its further definition as awareness-unity of limited truth; but the full basis for the outline is to be found in the relation of the various systems of truth to mind and in the various ways in which the content of awareness-unity is limited. Now an *x*, as that which is to be determined, implies something determined, an *abc*. As an outline or plan of that which is to be determined must be given, this outline is naturally included in the *abc*, though the detail to be filled in may fall within the *x*. In other words the outline, or at least an outline, belongs to the *abc* of psychology if psychology is to be defined at all. The *x* of psychology is, then, mind as the object to be determined on the basis of its outline or in the light of its fundamental structure. Given this outline or basic structure, research into the *x* can go forward systematically.

While the *x* would seem to be unlimited and inexhaustible to advancing knowledge, the outline as fundamental to the *x* is not so, because it includes only the beginning or foundation but not the detail of mental structure and function. Yet, in a study of the general outline as basic to the determination of the *x*, the definition of mind even if augmented by the addition of the forms of limitation of truth in relation to mind would not be sufficient to express the outline or lay the foundation. The foundation, therefore, must be more fully developed, and without encroaching upon the detail of mental truth. The definition of mind may and must give the clue to the outline; but without some building out of the outline, without clarification of the variety of problems it suggests, and without consideration of the direction or directions in which it leads and of the methods needed to advance into the *x*, no adequate foundation can be laid. The problem of the problem of psychology becomes the problem of the problems of psychology and the foundation must be the foundation of the problems. It must be not only the basis of the *x* but of the different groupings under which the *x* is to be brought, the various forms in which it is to be chiseled out.

Reference to the outline of the *x* as an *abc* and as the foundation of mental truth might make it seem as if the foundation were regarded as given, in the sense of being fixed and final, though the detail based upon it might change with advancing knowledge. Consequently it might seem as if the theory as to the foundation of mind offered in this work were to be regarded as absolute. However, it is not so intended. No theory is final but always subject to correction and alteration as knowledge moves forward. Even the logical core is subject to investigation and may be improved. The foundation of any science or field of knowledge may be relatively more stable than its detail, but it can never be final. Since the foundation and the detail dependent on it are interrelated, any augmentation of the detail or any advance to new levels or points of view may mean some readjustment in and overhauling of the foundation. Since this work is a study of the foundation, certain theories with regard to it are advanced and others rejected, but it is not intended that the theories advanced should be regarded as the last word. The foundation may condition the details to be determined, but the foundation as well as the detail is subject to alteration; and the theory pertaining to the foundation, like all theories, may be made over. The problem of the foundation, the problem of this work, whatever theory may be advanced with respect to it or however much may be done towards its solution, will remain always a problem and never become a finality.

If it be granted now that the outline is a foundation relative to the details to be determined and that it is a basis for the study of mind, it may be asked if it is the foundation of a system of mental truth. Does the psychological problem lead to a mental system just as the physical problem leads to a physical system, or the moral problem to a moral system? Undoubtedly a system of mental truth would be a looser system than a physical system and less unified than a moral system. A physical system hangs together as one vast causal nexus in space–time, and a moral system is grounded in a synthesis of all ends or all wills under definite principles. The mental world includes parts of the physical system, of the moral system, and of various other systems, as well as phases of the logical core, and so seems to be rather disjointed. Furthermore, it is limited, and also broken up into many separate and seemingly disconnected units or minds. Yet the study of mind may proceed in orderly fashion and systematically. The physical system is a system because it is based on order, and the same holds of the moral system. To the extent, then, to which mind might be handled in orderly fashion it might be said to be a system, so that while it may never be so perfect or articulate as the physical system, still, as based on an outline or foundation involving definite procedure in its determination, it may be regarded not merely as a region or world but as an order or system. Never self-sufficient but always dependent and limited, and involving a unique method for its determination, mind is nevertheless an object of systematic knowledge based on orderly procedure.

The outline of mind must now be developed as the foundation of the mental order. This outline is more than the definition of mind as given in the fundamental features of consciousness, yet it does not include the detail of mental truth. But it is dependent upon the definition and relative to the detail. Therefore, it must be built out on the basis of the definition and always with reference to the detail which it conditions. The definition as given in the four fundamental features of unity, awareness, content, and limitation of content was augmented by taking account of the relation of truth to mind as its content and of the various systems of truth which might have some place in the content. Two considerations must then be borne in mind, the fundamental features of mind and the relation of truth and the systems of truth to mind.

Of the fundamental features of mind or consciousness, unity taken by itself is insufficient to distinguish mind from anything else. In awareness, a distinguishing feature is to be found and combined with unity as awareness-unity; it forms the ground for the distinction between content and non-content. But awareness-unity would hardly be sufficient to suggest an outline; it merely marks off the field of mind. It is only in the content and the limitation of content that any adequate material suggestive of an outline can be found. The content, being made up of relations and phases of truth, is sufficiently complex to offer some basis for the outline and some differentiation within it. In the fundamental structure of truth, and also in the differentiation of the systems of truth as they appear in the content, such basis may be found. The limitation of content in its various forms has also something to offer. As it involves the grouping and massing of the content of consciousness in certain ways within awareness-unity it determines important factors in the outline. Thus, while unity and awareness are essential in defining mind, to develop the outline attention must be given both to the content as truth and to the forms of its limitation.

Truth with its structure and systems as content, and the forms or kinds of the limitation of content, when taken together offer a genuine clue as to the outline. They are taken together by considering the structure and systems of truth as content of awareness-unity under the forms of limitation. In other words, the structure and systems are determined so far as limited in the content of consciousness. The forms of limitation are imposed on truth, or it would be better to say that they are added to truth as further truth. This does not mean that truth with its structure and systems is interfered with or in any way disrupted. It is simply regrouped in consciousness and taken in a new but restricted setting. It is reshaped and reconstructed as it appears in consciousness and as within definite bounds. If the question is asked how a relation or a piece of truth's structure is grouped within the confines of the content of consciousness, the question is a question with regard to mental truth, a psychological question.

Before the outline is developed further three difficulties must be considered, difficulties with respect to mind and truth. First it may be asked, can mind include systematic truth? Secondly, can it include anything *but* systematic truth? Then, thirdly, it may be asked with regard to mind and truth, is not one the product of the other?

The first difficulty may be stated more expressly as follows: Truth being limited in consciousness, it might seem as if the structure and systems of truth, though not entirely disrupted, would be so disjointed and fragmentary in consciousness that they could never be really known by the mind. It might then be thought that the content of consciousness would consist merely of a flow or sequence of relations such that no structure or system of relations could ever appear in it. No truth but mental truth could be known, and objective truth, other than mental truth, would be hidden from the mind. Epistemological skepticism would then be in order.

The difficulty here stated can only be overcome by a consideration as to what objective truth is. Objective truth is orderly truth, and the mind tends to seek such truth. The beginning of order is to be found even in a relation. A relation has unity, specific connection, terms, and direction; that is, it has definite structure. A single relation taken by itself would not be sufficient to express a system of truth or a significant piece of truth's structure, but it does contain factors which suggest further relations. Direction is a factor which points beyond the relation itself; *a* and *b* being the terms of the relation, the direction from *a* to *b* suggests going on from *b* to *c* or to some other term thus leading beyond the original relation. Again, the terms of the relation may well be not only terminals of the original relation but relations themselves and terms of other relations, as the original relation itself may be a term in some other relation. Also, a multiple relation may suggest by its very structure the complexity of relations. With a group of relations possibly implied by a single relation the basis for order is laid. As all relations have structure, a mass or nexus of relations would naturally have structure and therefore exhibit order or system. Such order or system in the structure of relations makes possible objective truth or the order of relations in systems of truth. In all systems there are certain relations which are fundamental. They are called principles or postulates. There are all sorts of systems, relatively simple and relatively complex, important and unimportant, but there are certain fundamental systems to which most other systems reduce. Philosophy and science are concerned largely in filling out these fundamental systems, therefore they are for knowledge important systems. They have been classified in this work as imaginary, real, and teleological systems, with a logical core fundamental to them all. Now these systems and their sub-structures, including their fundamentals as well as their details, are food for the mind. They form its content and make up its object so far as they are orderly and systematic. The unity of their object lies in the unity or order of their structure or system. In contrast with the objective unity, the unity of the mind or awareness-unity never includes the full order and detail of the objective systems. But it can include some measure of objective truth and is not limited to a mere flow of relations. It includes objective truth either by grasping the outline of its order without filling in more than a minimum of its detail, or it takes in some phase of the order, some sub-structure with sufficient detail to suggest the beginning or at least a sign of order. As long as the mind aims at order, that is, attempts to seek the order of the content which appears, it aims at and even includes objective truth. In fact, not only does the mind seek an ordered object, but its content is made up of relations which imply structure and order. It is not then limited to passing relations but has access to the structure and systems of truth. The second difficulty appears once the first difficulty is overcome. It is the difficulty as to whether the content of the mind can include anything but systematic truth. If mind has access to the systems of truth, if the order and structure of truth can appear in its content, may it not be that all mental content is made up of systematic truth or at least of parts or phases of that truth? Mind's content would then be entirely objective.

Undoubtedly there is no content of consciousness which does not in some way have a place in systematic truth. The content is made up of relations, and these relations exhibit structure and order. They are, therefore, phases of systems or sub-systems themselves. The mind as including relations in its content can attempt to build out the structure or order into systems, to extend the order and fill in the detail. This procedure is unquestionably systematic, but even in content not recognized by the mind as belonging to any system or sub-system, in insignificant thoughts or in perceptions, the mind seeks structure or order, or, as is often said, it tries to make sense out of them. It may be baffled or fail in its attempt, but it always tries to grasp the connections and interrelationships among the details of its content. Yet the content is always fragmentary and partial. It is a phase or section of a system or structure; possibly it is a glimpse of the system outlined, but more commonly a group of subordinate relations; and the various phases and groupings are grasped sequentially and from various points of view by different minds. This fragmentary or partial character of the content cannot be accounted for by the systems of truth to which the relations in the content belong. A relation or a structure is not concerned with the manner in which it is grasped by minds. While, then, on the one hand no content can escape belonging to some objective structure, on the other hand it is limited and therefore subject to definite conditions. Consider the sum total of positive knowledge, the *abc,* the highest stage of truth which has been reached. It is not complete;

the *x* lies beyond it; but it includes all the systematic knowledge which is available. As a systematic structure or group of structures it does not as a whole fall within mind, but every relation or interrelation in it, every phase or aspect of it, either has fallen or does fall within some mind. Now the way it is spread out in minds, its distribution, is not a problem of positive knowledge so far as that knowledge is objective; it belongs to psychology or subjective knowledge. Again, the way in which positive knowledge or any part of it is spanned in consciousness and the way in which it flows or appears and disappears in consciousness are concerns not of objective knowledge but of psychology. Objective structures cannot fully define the mind or its content. In short, although all mental content belongs to a relational structure or objective system, the full truth about that content cannot be gathered from the structure or system to which it belongs.

Now as to the third difficulty. If systematic truth is included in mind and permeates its content but is not sufficient to determine it completely, may it not seem with regard to mind and systematic truth that one is at least the product of the other? It might be thought either that mind or at least it content results from some complexity or interrelationship of the objective systems of truth, or that the objective systems are creations or constructions of the mind.

If the former alternative is assumed, the mind might be regarded as the meeting point or intersection of the various systems, a sort of focus of objective truth. For instance, the moral world and the physical world affect each other at certain points. Mind might be the result or product of their interaction. Of course there can be no doubt as to the interplay of the objective systems in the content of consciousness, but it is very questionable whether consciousness or even the content of consciousness could be fully accounted for by such interplay. The limitation of the content and therefore of the interplay cannot be explained by the interplay itself. The way in which the structure of truth is packed in minds or mental compartments or distributed among these compartments is due to mind's structure rather than to the structure of the objective systems. Mind may be in part conditioned by objective truth, but it can hardly be said to follow from it or to be its creation.

According to the latter alternative, mind is thought not to be the cross-roads of the objective systems or in any way their product, but to be the producer of these systems. It is even thought to construct or actually fashion the systems, so that it may be regarded as the source of all truth. Positive knowledge, if not as a whole at least in all its parts, is included in the content of some mind or minds. Why not regard it, then, as of mind's own making? But if it were mind-made, truth would not stand on its own feet. Many idealists have accepted such a view, but the difficulty involved can be easily overcome. The mind may contain truth within itself, that is, include truth within its content; it may select details of truth or set up postulates; but the details or postulates are true because they fit into the systems of truth, not because they belong to mind. Though the mind may attend to certain truths, those truths are not due to the mind. It may take a mind to formulate the law of action and reaction, or to map out the solar system, but both the law and the map hold relatively to the system in which they have their place. It is a fundamental misconception to assume that logical truth or real truth or even the truth of imaginary or teleological systems is a creation of the mind. The content of awareness-unity is truth made up of relations belonging to various systems; but its being content does not mean that it is primarily content, hence in origin mind, and only secondarily truth, a resultant or deposit of mind. However closely mind may be bound up with truth, truth as structure and system cannot be said to be its product.

A consideration of the method of reconstruction used in psychology may throw further light on the relation of mind to objective truth. Knowledge moves forward step by step, from one stage of truth to another; the *abc* encroaches on the *x* of truth and knowledge, thereby determining more and more. This procedure is objective, it is the constructive method of philosophy and science. In psychology, as in other branches of knowledge, the constructive method is used, but because of the relation of objective truth to the mind, the objective truth being the matter of the content of consciousness, the method of psychology is, more correctly speaking, a *re*-constructive method. It is a resetting or reconstructing of truth as relative to mental limitations, or an interpreting of mind on the basis of already constructed objective knowledge. It either reconstructs truth to determine mind or it reconstructs mind by way of truth. But whether as reconstruction of truth or of mind it is *re*-construction because it is dependent on prior construction. Construction means making, building, or forming, and the theories and syntheses of science are often spoken of as made or constructed by the scientific mind. To regard scientific constructions as literally made or formed by the mind has the advantage of warding off the view that the truths of science are given and already there to be found by merely looking at things, instead of being suggested by the imagination. They may be the product and creation of imagination, but however fertile the imagination may be in producing them its main function in knowledge is to suggest the possible ways in which the relations of truth may hang together, to fit the various theories into the structures and systems of truth. Construction in knowledge refers much more to this fitting together of truth than it does to the productive power of imagination. So understood, construction means putting together as interpreting or construing. The constructions of science are the interpretations and ways of construing truth as knowledge advances. Reconstruction is then a reinterpretation or further interpretation, a construing on the basis of something already construed, a reconstruing. If now the method of construction is not a method of making truth but of construing or interpreting it, it ought to be clear that truth is not a product of the imagination or of mind but is something holding in its own right and fundamentally independent of mind. And if the method of reconstruction is not a remaking the mind or a making over of objective truth into mind, but is an interpretation of the mind, that is, a reinterpreting or reconstruing of objective truth as relative to mind in order to interpret mind, it ought also to be clear that mind, though understood through the mediation of objective truth, is not its product.

Construction and reconstruction are then both methods of interpretation, the one primary and the other secondary. Therefore, they are not methods of forming and fashioning something but methods of determining what objective truth and mind are. The view that the constructions of knowledge are the product of the creative activity of the mind, and that the mind can only be known by a reconstruction of its nature on the basis of the study of its creations, presupposes the conception of construction as production and of reconstruction as an attempt to get back to the source of construction. Here reconstruction is not taken as a kind of secondary production based on the primary objective production or construction but rather as an interpretation of mind. Construction and reconstruction are used in two different senses, and strictly speaking the only object to be determined is the object or subject, mind, objective truth being fundamentally only the revelation of mind. Such a view leads to a very narrow idealism or mentalism. It cannot hold if truth is to have any status of its own. It is important, then, to be consistent in conceiving of the methods of construction and reconstruction and to regard them as methods for interpreting and determining the nature of objective truth and mind.

With due consideration for the difficulties here mentioned in connection with the relation of mind to truth, it is now possible to work out the outline of mind. The outline of mind is mind's skeletal structure and the foundation of all mental truth. It therefore defines the object of psychological investigation. The method used by psychology, that of reconstruction, is also determined by this outline. As was said above, the two principal considerations involved in outlining mind are the systems of truth and the forms of limitation of consciousness. As mind is made up of the structure and systems of truth as the content of awareness-unity subject to limitations, the lines and general forms of truth as limited content must be defined by some combination of these lines and forms. This combination can be effected by considering the lines of truth suggested by its systems as falling under the forms of limitation. That is, the outline of mind consists of the lines of truth in relation to and subordinate to the forms of limitation. To make the outline clear the forms of limitation with the lines of truth falling under them must be made explicit. To state the matter in terms of method the systems of truth must be reconstructed with reference to the forms of limitation. The further elucidation of this skeleton of mind must now be undertaken.

To make clear the outline on the basis of the combination mentioned it will be necessary to consider the various systems of truth as they fall under the different forms of limitation. The systems of truth as already classified will be sufficient for the outline, but the forms of limitation must be stated once more. Its four fundamental forms or kinds have been mentioned in Chapter IV. First of all, there is the limitation of the span of consciousness in one awareness-unity. This includes both the span of perception and the span of imagination, suggesting respectively the limitation of the present and the limitation of the given. Secondly, there is the limitation connected with the change of the content of consciousness. Factors in the content appear, but they also disappear and their disappearance marks a limitation. All content being in flux, much is lost; and that which is gained must be caught on the wing. Thirdly, the division of the factors in the content is limited. It is not possible to break up these factors beyond a certain point, as, for instance, in the case of a vague feeling or the quality of a sensation. Fourthly, there is the limitation of the individual consciousness. Not only are there the individual differences in perception and imagery, but also the differences in the various points of view of truth relative to the different individual consciousnesses, truth never having a sufficient expression in any one mind. In brief, the content of awareness-unity is limited in extension, by loss of detail because in flux, in division of detail, and by being scattered in various individual minds. Under these fundamental forms the lines or systems of truth must be ranged.

As for the substance of the outline, it would seem natural to begin by showing how the most fundamental and therefore the most universal side of systematic truth falls under the forms of limitation, and then to go on to the less universal side, the different systems of truth, and as far as possible in the order of their universality. This procedure means consideration, first of the logical core, then of the imaginary systems, and after that of the real and teleological systems.

The first consideration is to show how the forms of limitation work relatively to the logical core, how they bring about certain mental functions or phenomena in connection with logical truth as content. The most universal character of logical truth, and for that matter of all truth, is that it is synthetic, connected, or relational. As all truth consists of relations, it might be pertinent before considering the logical relations to ask whether any or all relations, so far as they fall within the limitations of the content of mind, give rise to any phenomenon or form of massing in consciousness occasioned by the limitations. There is one phenomenon which appears in connection with relations as content, that is, the phenomenon of attention. The content of consciousness always appears with some of the relations in it or phases of it stressed and emphasized more than others, with the central part of its area or field standing out more clearly and intensely than the other parts and forming a sort of center or focal point in the content. This clear and central portion of the content is often conceived of as the part attended to by the mind as if the mind included some agency over and above its content, but such a conception is inaccurate, as all agencies of the mind belong to the content. It would be more correct to bring out the phenomenon of attention by referring merely to the content of consciousness as massed in such a way that it would contain a central part which is clearer than the other parts. Attention should first of all be defined on the basis of clearness in the mental field. True, attention is closely connected with the selection of ends or purposes as the basis of practical activities, but it is also, and in a more fundamental way, a phase of the massing of relations in consciousness. It should furthermore be pointed out that attention is constantly shifting, or better, that the relations forming the clear and central part of the content are always changing. Even when the mind is trying to grasp a single relation, the relation is not taken in evenly and all at once, the different factors in it being stressed and attended to in succession. It might now seem as if the phenomenon of attention were not due to the forms of limitation of content. It is quite easy to imagine a limited field with all its detail equally clear. Such a field would be limited but would not contain the phenomenon of attention. So far as the limitation of the span of consciousness goes, attention would not seem to be necessary. With the limitation connected with change in content the situation is different. Of the relations which appear in and disappear from the content of consciousness, some disappear less quickly and are retained relatively longer than others. For those that remain longer greater clearness is possible and attention may be given to them. Again, any striving to make certain factors clear would tend to make them remain longer as content. In other words, attention or the clearness of some part of the content is a counterpoise to the limitation connected with change or the passing of content out of consciousness, and it is also in some measure due to this limitation or at least conditioned by it. Thus attention would seem to be occasioned by one of the fundamental forms of limitation.

As suggested above, selection plays a part in attention. It might be said to spring from the interest of the mind in certain details for practical or other purposes. It is, of course, limited by the first two fundamental forms of limitation, since it cannot select factors not included in the content or which have not entered the content, although the mind may strive to include factors not already included. The phenomenon of attention may then be said to include both clearness and selection of content, clearness being more fundamental. Both features appear in connection with the forms of limitation and are involved in the massing and grouping of content in consciousness.

Now as to the logical relations, those fundamental to truth.

In Chapter IV, in discussing the question how a limited mind may know logical principles, it was pointed out that concepts and judgments were special forms or ways in which consciousness includes truth within its content. Concept and judgment, with their extension in inference and reasoning, are the mental forms in which much truth is expressed; and they are most decidedly the forms in which logical truth gets its expression in consciousness. Of these forms judgment is primary and fundamental. It appears as basic to concepts, percepts, feelings, and in all content in which there is a recognition of the relation of one relation to another or to a group of relations. Judgment as well as the other forms are necessitated by the limitations of content. Just as with attention, if logical relations or all truth could be given directly and in one unity of consciousness, judgment would not be needed; but with the limitations due to span and change some form of apprehending and recognizing relations and interrelations as given in content, and before they disappear from it, is required. Judgment and attention, then, are both essential in apprehending logical relations; attentive judgment is necessary to bring the logical core within the range of mind. As a result, attention, involving both clearness and selection, and judgment with its associates, concept, reasoning, percept, etc., suggest the primary features in the outline of mind.

The method of reconstruction is here involved. It ought to be obvious that judgment and attention cannot be gotten at directly. It is necessary to start with objective truth or relations and then to see that the form in which they appear in mind, the form in which they are massed in consciousness, can be gotten at only by reconstruing the objective truth as relative to consciousness. The object must be determined as content of a narrow and flowing consciousness after the structure of the object has been determined. Quite clearly, in large groups of relations, or in the complexity of a relational structure, the relational group or structure comes first and the way it is explored by limited consciousness is secondary. And not only do the span of consciousness and the change of consciousness limit the mental grasp of such group or structure, but the limitation in the division of content also plays its part. Mental analysis and penetration into the detail of a structure cannot go beyond a certain point. Then, too, in the building up of knowledge there is a division of labor. No one mind can grasp it all; different minds conceive different parts of it and contribute in different ways to its development. All four forms of limitation play their part in determining the outline which is gotten at by a kind of fundamental reconstruction basic to psychological research.

With the rather meagre statement given above as to the phases of the outline suggested by the logical core, the more special systems must now be considered. Imaginary systems help little in adding to the outline, except possibly by bringing out more fully the character of selection in attention. Imaginary systems are systems devised to meet problems appearing in the field of imagination. A six-dimensional space, a purely ideal moral world, and a reality other than that connected with the physical or mental worlds, as well as incomplete or inconsistent spheres, would be examples of such systems. It would be quite possible to start with certain relations which seem to involve six dimensions and then to ask what the conditions of a six-dimensional system would be. Or it would be possible to start by setting up certain postulates and then carrying out the system which these postulates condition. In either case the systems could be true systems, systems of objective truth, but they would be somewhat arbitrarily chosen. They might not have much value, but they would express regions of truth, having their place in truth along with truth more vital and more significant to human interest. But they would not help to define some fundamental phase or function of the human mind. As the principles of these systems, unlike the logical core, would not condition all truth, they might be chosen rather freely and treated as, so to speak, systems *ad libitum*. As far as the outline of mind goes this would only help to bring out the phenomenon of selection a little more fully, as it might also suggest the range of the imagination. Otherwise imaginary systems have little or nothing to offer in bringing out the mental outline.

The real and teleological systems yield more. The question at once arises as to which of the two should be considered first. It is more usual to consider the real before the ideal, but as the ideal or teleological truth has greater sweep than real truth, since it involves both the real and the ideal, it will here be considered first.

In this work teleological problems and systems have been divided into moral, aesthetic, and technical. The moral system is the most universal in that it includes all ends and all wills as willing ends. It is concerned with the final and complete goal of all purpose, therefore it should be regarded as more fundamental than the technical and aesthetic spheres, and it is indeed unusually helpful in reconstructing the outline of mind. The moral ideal or unity or law is the condition of the moral system, and as such is the basis of moral truth. It is also the goal or end of all moral activity. It is, then, both truth and end. But in including more specific ends it includes the wills willing those ends and it includes the original germs or tendencies motivating those ends. Not only is it truth and end but it involves will and motive. These four features of the moral system are all distinguished within it as fundamental phases of its objective truth, and when brought under the forms of limitation they determine the outline in various ways.

So far as moral truth goes, it falls within the limitations of mind just as any truth does in the form of judgment and concept and with the aid of attention. Though as expressing moral principle it may seem to expand the ideal to its utmost as well as to include the real, it is conceived by the mind without the aid of any superior function. Moral principle as an end, however, implies movement and progression, an incorporating of the ideal in the real. Progression brings with it two features: the goal aimed at or to be attained, and the moving reality moving towards the goal; that is, the not yet determined but to be determined, and the determining activity with that which has been determined. In this double process the essence of teleology is expressed. As brought under the limitations of content of mind, process is narrowed down by the second fundamental limitation, that due to change. The moving reality is largely a present reality, and the goal or that which is to be determined is limited by the span of the imagination. The distinction between the given and the present, between the not yet determined and the determined, between the ideal and real as content of consciousness, appears at this point, and it should be noted that the distinction is based on objective considerations. The will or volition is the self-direction of the mind, and self-direction is, more specifically, (a) idea and (b) act based on idea. Now the idea falls within the given as a possible goal, and the act based on it takes place in the present. Both the idea and the act involve attention, which is of vital importance in selecting the end and in making the decision to act. The series of ends or ideas selected and the series of decisions made make up the nucleus of the moral individual or person. This moral individual or individual will is the unit of the moral system of wills, and as a mental unit falls under the fourth fundamental limitation, that of individual consciousness. The moral system first defines the moral person or the moral agent as moral, the mental limitation of distinct persons with the various features connected with these persons in the content of consciousness being secondary. Furthermore, the motive which leads will in one direction or another, which connects it with specific ends, is the material element in the moral system. It might be called tendency, or desire, or material end. This factor stands out in the moral system by contrast with the synthesis or unity of all ends, and is often spoken of as an interest or inclination; it is that which gives character and directs toward particular ends. When taken account of in reconstruction of mind, it appears as something which cannot be further analyzed and broken up, and therefore as conditioned by the third fundamental limitation.

The features important to the outline which result from the consideration of the moral system, beside judgment and attention, are, then, first, the tying down to the present of the transforming of the ideal into the real, the distinction between the given and the present, idea and act as based on that which is to be determined and on the determining – in other words, that which is fundamental to will; second, desire or tendency or material end as contrasted with the synthesis and order of ends and as the original factor in motivation. The same result may be reached by considering technical systems, systems concerned with finding the means necessary to the attainment of ends. Instead of the synthesis of all ends there would be an end which would define and unify the means to the attainment of that end. But the mental factors of judgment, attention transforming the ideal into the real, distinguishing the present from the given, material elements or desire, and the various features connected with the will, are the same. Any teleological system might be sufficient to bring out the various factors related to the will in consciousness. Even the aesthetic object has little more to suggest unless possibly the factor of feeling. An aesthetic object may seem to imply a certain unity, perfection, or finish, and it may also be in some way an expression of human nature. So far, however, as a feeling of pleasure might be said to accompany the contemplation of the aesthetic object, pleasure may be said to appear as an unanalyzable factor and something which cannot further be broken up within the limits of mind. Unquestionably, whether the moral, technical, or aesthetic side of teleological truth be considered, the limited content of mind includes something teleological and purposive in its outline.

Now as to the physical system, it should be pointed out that as brought under the limitations of content it is primarily an object or objective system, to be known by the mind. As known it involves judgment and attention and it includes very varied detail, detail often spoken of as empirical truth. The physical system is the space–time system, and the mind would seem to be in closest touch with it in perception; but if it were limited to perception the mind would have no adequate view of it as a system. Not only is there perception of the physical world but there is also conception of it, both perception and conception presupposing judgment. As perception is limited to the present no adequate conception of the system could be attained without the help of the imagination. The imagination, so important in teleological consideration, is here essential in grasping the past and in forecasting the future, and also in taking in those phases of the system not touched by perception. In perception two important features appear, extension and duration. Objects are perceived in spatial and temporal order. But now, if it be asked, what is there that appears in perception which is not the spatial and temporal order or arrangement of the objects, that is, what is it that is arranged or ordered? the answer would be, sensations or the material factor in perception. The physical system then suggests for the content of mind concept, percept, imagination, the space and time order, and sensation. These must be considered relative to the limitations of the content of mind.

Of all the mental functions, concepts have the widest range, often covering detail not included in the content of consciousness. It is on the basis of concepts that the mind stretches out to wider and wider perspectives of truth. By means of them it may include not only the postulates of the physical system but also principles covering empirical detail. But it is limited to the given in its actual application, the given or total content of consciousness marking the limit of imagination. The imagination is of the utmost importance to mind in grasping the physical world, particularly in grasping the past and future and in distinguishing them from the present. Its wide range is due largely to the change and movement of its content rather than to its span. Though it is by no means so limited in span as perception, its limitation is significant for concepts, since their detail is suggested by its content. The alteration in its content is a kind of sequence of objective content, a flow of objects, and as such it is a sequence which cannot be entirely reduced to the space–time order. The span of perception is much more limited than that of imagination. Its spatial extension is sometimes considerable, but its temporal expansion is very small, varying from a small fraction of a second to about six seconds. It is a mistake to suppose that the temporal span in perception is what is commonly called the "specious present" involving the continuing and gradual disappearing of factors appearing in perception.[1] The continuing and gradual disappearing of the factors is not vital to the span, it is primarily a grasping of a piece of time, an awareness-unity of a bit of what Whitehead, in his account of the act of becoming, calls "temporal extension." [2] The flow of perception is essentially spatio-temporal, as is also the imagery of the imagination. But now it should not be supposed that there are two separate worlds of sequence. The flow of the content of consciousness is in a sense one stream, but much of its objective sequence cannot be reduced to space–time sequence, though the sequence of objective content may include temporal sequences. This simply means not only that consciousness and its content, but also the sequence and flow of its content, cannot be fully absorbed by the space–time system. Then, in contrast with the barriers of the mind found in the span of consciousness and the flow of its content, its lower limit should not be forgotten. Sensation like desire and feeling represents this lower limit and is a fundamental feature in perception. In fact, perception would not be perception without sensation, although perception is not merely a group of sensations. Sensation is a kind of final factor in the detail of the content of consciousness and can be conceived only through reconstruction. Though knowledge seems to get its expression in the mind primarily in concepts and ideas based on judgment, it is still very closely bound up with and limited by imagination, perception, and sensation, and with their content both as given and as changing.

The outline of mind can now be stated more briefly and more compactly. It is based on the definition of mind as consciousness or as awareness-unity of limited content, the content being made up of truth. As unity and awareness offer no differentiating marks within consciousness, the study

[1] Howard Crosby Warren, *Human Psychology* (Boston and New York, 1919), p. 255.

[2] Alfred North Whitehead, *Process and Reality* (Cambridge, 1929), p. 107.

of mind comes down to a study of the limited content or of truth as content and as brought under the forms of limitation. The various lines of truth as relative to the forms of limitation suggest the primary character of the outline. The problem of psychology is to determine how the structures or the systems of truth are compacted within the confines of the content of mind. Truth and its systems of relations as limited by the limitations of span, change, division, and plurality of centers appear in mind under the following forms:

1. (a) Attention. The relations of truth are so massed in the content of consciousness that the central part of the content is clearer than the other parts and with the relations falling within this part is constantly changing. (b) Judgment. The relations and interrelations appearing and attended to are recognized and assented to as true. (c) Plurality of conscious centers. Truth is massed in many apparently distinct consciousnesses, in individual conscious centers.

2. The relations of truth are so massed that will or self-direction of the mind is possible. Will involves: (a) selection, by means of attention, of ideas as ideals or ends to be realized, ends, moral, technical, or aesthetic, and (b) the realization of ideals or ends only in the present, the distinction between the given and the present being involved; and will includes (c) individual wills, the plurality of teleological or purposive consciousnesses.

3. Physical truth is massed in consciousness with the aid of attention and judgment, and in many conscious centers, but under certain further conditions: (a) Concepts or the fixed grasping of relations both fundamental and empirical are needed to give foundation and substance to knowledge. (b) Percepts are necessary as a way of grasping the detail of the present. (c) Imagination with its images is necessary as including all non-present detail, past, future, etc. (d) Change of content both as temporal change and as the sequence of objective content is an essential condition affecting the change of concepts, percepts, and images and the development and growth of knowledge.

4. There is a final irreducible factor involved in the mass-

ing of truth in the mind. This is the material element—desire, feeling, and sensation.

Such is the outline of mind, the skeleton of mind's content. Mind turns out to be a plurality of consciousnesses, each consciousness having an attending, judging, willing, conceiving, imagining, perceiving, desiring, sensing, feeling, and changing content. It is for the psychologists to determine this content, that is, to carry out the forms and functions here given and to fill in the detail of the structure outlined. The outline seems to include four phases which might be referred to roughly as thinking, willing, knowing, and the material element. It should, of course, not be supposed that the mind is made up of separate parts or that the phases of the outline refer to distinct faculties or powers. Nor does the old division of consciousness into "knowing, willing, and feeling" have any value except as it reflects objective truth. The different phases of the outline represent different lines or strata of truth as it appears in consciousness.

The first phase of the outline, thinking, includes the consciousness of truth and its relations so far as its fundamental structure and development are concerned. Clearness of thought, judgment and reasoning, selection of ideas, and the division of labor among minds in the pursuit of knowledge are here involved, and they form the basis for the study of attention, judgment, discrimination, analysis, synthesis, conception, inference, meaning, and the suggestion and interchange of ideas as mental functions. Fundamental relations suggested by the study of logic and in part of imaginary systems would come into play. The study of this phase of the mind is almost a study by itself, and it is basic to the comprehension of the other phases. Its central problem might be said to be the problem of the consciousness of object or of the primary mental functions involved in thinking objective truth.

The second phase, willing, includes the teleological side of consciousness, the consciousness of ends, purposes, or ideals and their realization. It is the basis for the study of moral, technical, and aesthetic ideals, including the study of value, interest, taste, character, personality, individuals in their relation to one another, distinction between the given and the present, and the process of self-direction and realization. This side of the mind which is concerned with the development of wills, persons, or selves cannot be studied entirely in separation from the rest of mind, but it forms a very important chapter in psychology.

The third phase, knowing, covers consciousness or its content so far as it is suggested or conditioned by the physical system. The distinction between conception, imagination, and perception stands out in this phase of the outline, as also the feature of change both as temporal change and as sequence of objective content. There is much detail to be worked out in connection with conception, with imagination and its imagery, and with the various forms of perception. But the feature of change is by far the most vital, radical, and far-reaching problem suggested by this phase of the outline. It is not the problem of how the content changes in time; it is rather the problem of how time and change appear in consciousness.

The fourth phase includes the material element. Desire, feeling, and sensation are or at least include irreducible factors which appear in connection with volition and perception. They are part of the filling of the content of mind which cannot be entirely identified with these other functions. Desire as tendency or direction, feelings of pleasure and displeasure, and the whole scale of sensations offer material for special study even if the result of that study yields little more than a classification of these material elements.

Though the detail to be supplied in the outline is extensive, it centers in four fundamental problems, the problem of the basis of the objective, of the teleological, of time and change, and of the irreducible elements as they appear in the content of mind. The structure of truth is crucial in defining this grouping of problems. But a somewhat different grouping might be made by giving greater emphasis to the forms of limitation. First, by consideration of the span of consciousness, the general structure of the given might be studied.

Conception, imagination, perception, including the conception and perception of time and space as well as everything embraced in the general area of the content, would here be dealt with. It would be a kind of structural psychology, concerned with the general make-up of the content. Then, secondly, by consideration of the change of content study could be made of the growth of knowledge and mind, the self-direction of the mind in will, the spontaneity of the imagination, the realization of ideals, the development of personality, and of time and change itself as fundamental to all other functions. This would be a kind of functional psychology concerned with the functions of the mind in a changing content. In the third place, the lower limit of mind could be studied, consideration being given to the various kinds of irreducibles. Here a classification of sensations would be in order, as also a study of desire in its relation to emotion, instinct, feeling, etc., including possibly a study of formal irreducibles such as difference and unity. Finally, the individual consciousness could be studied as the basis for the relation of the individual units to one another. This would be social psychology. Animal psychology might even be included here, as also the problem of the so-called "sub-conscious" mind as possibly consisting of lower but separate centers of consciousness. The particular way, however, in which the features of the outline are grouped is of less consequence than the features themselves, their interrelations, and their place and function in the mental structure.

To understand the outline is to understand the layout of mind's content as truth under limitations. Both truth and the limitations define this content, but truth is primary and the limitations secondary. Therefore, the method of determining the content is that of reconstruction. The method of external observation, of observing the behavior of organisms, yields nothing but an account of behavior and never leads to consciousness unless the description is taken as a sign or suggestion of a conscious content which must be reconstructed on the basis of known truth or content. And the method of introspection is insufficient because whatever is observed directly as content of consciousness can only be understood in the light of a larger conception of mind than can be acquired on the basis of immediate observation. Introspection is at its best in analyzing the irreducible factors in the content. But even in its analysis, for instance, of sensation, it presupposes perception, which is itself a kind of objectification, the sensation as an irreducible element being brought out by reconstruction. The introspective method is primarily a method of analysis, and since analysis is of value as a preliminary to synthesis, this method is a deficient one or at best only a phase of a fuller method. As truth is synthetic, the truth about mind is synthetic, and the study of mind implies a synthetic method. Truth consists of relations, therefore psychology is the psychology of relations, its object, the content of mind, consisting of truth and hence of relations. The *Gestalt* psychology so well explained by Köhler [3] comes nearer than any of the other psychologies of today to the type of psychology consistent with the outline here advocated. The reconstructive method can never be coupled with the causal method of explanation. To explain mind causally would mean to fit it into the physical system. The content of mind is only partially conditioned by the physical system, therefore the causal method is only of limited value. As mind includes truth from several systems, not merely from the causal system, all those systems condition and explain its content. Mental truth is objective truth reorganized and reconstrued as limited content of mind; that is, it is reconstructed truth.

The question might here naturally arise as to whether mental truth is not objective truth. It is objective truth in the sense that it is valid or binding truth, in other words, true truth. The only reason for regarding non-mental truth as objective, and contrasting mental truth with it as subjective and hence not objective, is to be found in the secondary character of mental truth and in its dependence on non-mental truth. On the basis of the constructions of non-mental or objective truth, mental truth is reconstructed. Though it is dependent truth, it is just as true as any other truth. The

[3] Wolfgang Köhler, *Gestalt Psychology* (New York, 1929), pp. 187–223.

system of mental truth has its place, though a unique place, in the whole body of truth. Moreover, the attempt of mind to conceive itself, to know mental truth, is an attempt to get at the mental order just as it might attempt to get at the physical order or moral order, and while the determination of itself may involve a more complicated method, it is an object conceived like any other object within the mental content. Philosophers might avoid confusion by referring to non-mental truth as objective and by referring to mental truth as both objective and subjective.

A possible objection may be made to the whole theory of psychology here advocated. It may be said that the kind of psychology suggested and defined in this work seems little like the psychology or psychologies which are being developed today. It may be said to be out of tune with psychological research. By way of making the objection more definite it may be claimed that the psychology of this work is vague, unsystematic, and unscientific. If psychology is regarded as the study of mind as conditioned by and as explained by reference to the nervous system, or if it is regarded simply as behavior unified through the nervous system, then it is unlike the psychology here advocated. This work is in a sense a protest against the neural explanation of mind and against regarding mind as merely behavior. It maintains that mind is primarily consciousness, and that psychology as the science of mind is the science of consciousness. The study of the neural conditions of mind and behaviorism are both, strictly speaking, branches of biology. If the former is concerned with content, which seems to lie close to mind, and if the latter studies functions once thought of as mental, they might be considered as a kind of psychological biology or biological psychology, but as they are not concerned directly with the core of things mental or psychical, they can hardly be regarded as branches of psychology proper. This work is, however, not out of tune with many of the older psychologies and those of the present day which emphasize consciousness and make it central in their study. It is in fact an attempt to get at the presuppositions of just this kind of psychology. As for any claim that the psychology of this work is vague, it is undoubtedly true that mind as consciousness is a much more subtle and difficult thing to grasp than many other kinds of objects. Just as physiology might be said to be a vaguer science than arithmetic because it involves a greater number and variety of conceptions, so psychology as a science of consciousness might be said to be vaguer than any other branch of knowledge because it is dependent on almost all branches of knowledge and so involves a far greater variety of conceptions. But the fact that the conception of consciousness presupposes so much and is difficult to bring before the mind is no ground for claiming that consciousness is not the true object of psychology or could not be determined by an appropriate method. Then, as to the claim that this psychology is unsystematic, it ought to be clear from what has been said earlier in this chapter that mind as consciousness can be determined by systematic procedure, though the procedure may be complex. Because mind includes parts and phases of various objective systems of truth it cannot be regarded as something indefinite and elusive and therefore itself not a system. The definition of mind, its relation to the systems of objective truth, and the outline of its content offer a foundation for its orderly and methodical determination. As following orderly procedure in the determination of its object, psychology is systematic; and as systematic it may be referred to as a science. The kernel of the objection seems to lie in the claim that this psychology is unscientific. A body of knowledge resulting from the determination of an object or system of truth by orderly procedure is generally referred to as a science. At the same time the term *science* is regarded by many as the equivalent of natural science, that is, the term *science* is limited to those sciences which are concerned with the physical world or any part of it. In the theory of mind developed in this work mind is not regarded as a physical object; consequently psychology is not a physical science. It would, then, according to the narrower conception of science, not be a science at all. No doubt the accuracy of causal explanation, the relative clearness of sequences in space–time open to everyone's observation, and the fact that observations and experiments can be more easily verified in physical science than in other regions have made many feel that only in physical science is there the accuracy and opportunity for verification which make possible scientific as opposed to non-scientific knowledge. The question here is the question as to whether science includes all systematic knowledge or only such systematic knowledge as is reducible to the physical system and amenable to the methods of natural science. It is a question of completeness of knowledge versus the accuracy of natural science. To look askance at psychology and other branches of knowledge which have not the accuracy of natural science and to label them as unscientific is unfortunate. A prejudice in favor of natural science tends to put the center of gravity of truth in the physical system and to reduce all truth to physical truth, thus throwing the whole system of knowledge out of balance. But the difficulty may be overcome if the non-physical branches of knowledge are allowed the status of sciences on condition that they exhibit as high a degree of accuracy as the objects which they seek to determine permit. Each branch, then, according to the character of its object, but each a science if it determines its object methodically. Accordingly, it would seem appropriate to refer to the psychology of consciousness as a science.

Psychology as a science may then have its place in the system of sciences just as mind is thought of as having its place in the system of truth. The possibility of a science of mind has been established in these pages by developing an outline of mind on the basis of the relation of mind to truth, the outline defining the field to be investigated. To develop this outline it was necessary to consider both truth and mind and then the relation of mind to truth. In accordance with the relational theory of truth, truth was shown to consist of relations, of a system or structure of relations centering in a core of fundamental relations. This system was shown to run out into various sub-systems, logical, imaginary, real, and teleological. The system or sub-systems were not regarded as expressing final or absolute truth, as it was found impossible to determine the structure of any ultimate system of things, nor were they thought of as in any way mental or as produced by mind, though mind might know them. Truth was rather to be considered as a developing structure, moving along from stage to stage. This dynamic aspect of truth was spoken of as its second dimension, the dimension of knowledge. Positive knowledge, knowledge actually determined, could only be a perspective of truth, a structure of relations at a particular stage. This whole theory of truth was developed along the lines of logical idealism and of a restricted form of epistemological idealism. Mind was then considered. Three theories of mind were criticized — behaviorism, the content theory, and the ego–content theory. Behaviorism was shown to be inadequate and insufficient to account for the phenomena of consciousness, and the content theory, though a theory of mind as consciousness, was shown to have too narrow a conception of consciousness and to be in danger of having to explain mind by brain function. The ego–content theory was modified by leaving out the ego but by retaining the functions of unity and awareness over and above content. As a result, an awareness-unity theory of mind was accepted, and mind was defined as an awareness-unity of limited content, unity, awareness, content, and its limitation being the four fundamental features of mind and all essential to its definition. In this connection it was brought out that the reconstructive method of description was more appropriate to the awareness-unity theory of mind than the method of introspection or that of external observation, although these two methods might be used as aids to reconstruction. It was also brought out that a non-causal system of explanation was involved, as neither consciousness nor its content could be brought entirely within the space–time or causal system. After the consideration of truth and mind, the relation of mind to truth was taken up. Mind and truth were seen to be related in two fundamental ways. On the one hand, mind as an object of truth was shown to have its place in the system of truth, as one of truth's sub-systems, and therefore to be an addendum to non-mental or objective truth. On the other hand, truth was shown to have a place in mind, its relational structure — at least part of it — forming the content of consciousness. Mind was then redefined as the awareness-unity of limited truth, as truth massed and grouped within the confines of consciousness, such truth belonging primarily to the objective systems of truth and secondarily to the content. Unity and awareness, however important they might be in binding together the content and in distinguishing the content from non-content, were seen to offer no distinguishing marks internal to mind; consequently it was made clear that the detail and varying features of mind were to be found only in truth as its content and in the limitations of the content. The four fundamental forms of limitation found in (a) span, (b) change, and (c) division of content, and in (d) plurality of minds, and the various lines and systems of truth, were considered as the determining features of the outline of mind and its content. The relation of the various systems of truth to mind was given careful consideration, their influence on its content as restricted by the forms of limitation being emphasized. Then the outline or skeleton of mind was brought out by grouping its fundamental features under the functions of thinking, willing, knowing, and the material element, special emphasis being laid on logical, moral, and physical truth in shaping the outline. Finally, it was shown on the basis of the outline how the detail of mind could be determined by the reconstructive and non-causal method, reconstructive because based on the prior construction of objective systems of truth and non-causal because based on several objective systems and not solely on the physical system. Thus it was made clear that the lines of psychological research and the appropriate psychological method were centered in and determined by the outline of mind.

The *x* of psychology, the object to be determined in psychological investigation, mind, has now been defined and outlined. It has been distinguished from and contrasted with other objects of study, and a method has been suggested for its determination. The problem of the problem of psychology has thus been clarified, or at least progress towards its clarification has been made. The problem of psychology has been set though it has not been solved, since the detail of the object outlined has not been filled in or determined. The way has been devious and has involved the survey of the whole field of knowledge from a philosophical point of view. The theories and views expressed are concerned solely with establishing the foundation or presuppositions of psychology. The work is philosophical, not psychological. It will probably not satisfy many psychologists, yet it offers a unique place to psychology in the system of knowledge, a place which cannot be filled by any other science or branch of knowledge and which is needed to round out the whole structure of knowledge and truth.

INDEX

Bei Fragen zur Produktsicherheit wenden Sie sich bitte an:
If you have any questions regarding product safety,
please contact:

Walter de Gruyter GmbH
Genthiner Straße 13
10785 Berlin
productsafety@degruyterbrill.com